Antimicrobial Coatings for Biodegradable Polymers

Antimicrobial Coatings for Biodegradable Polymers:

The Medical Nanorevolution

By

Iva Rezić

Cambridge Scholars Publishing

Antimicrobial Coatings for Biodegradable Polymers:
The Medical Nanorevolution

By Iva Rezić

This book first published 2023

Cambridge Scholars Publishing

Lady Stephenson Library, Newcastle upon Tyne, NE6 2PA, UK

British Library Cataloguing in Publication Data
A catalogue record for this book is available from the British Library

ISBN (10): 1-5275-3648-3
ISBN (13): 978-1-5275-3648-7

To Jure and Ernest

TABLE OF CONTENTS

PREFACE

In an era where the relentless march of science and technology shapes the contours of our world, the realm of medicine and healthcare stands as a testament to the remarkable progress humanity has achieved. Yet, amid these strides towards healthier lives, a persistent challenge continues to cast a shadow on our achievements – the escalating threat of antimicrobial resistance. As we grapple with the evolution of pathogens that defy conventional treatments, the need for innovative and effective solutions has never been more pressing.

This book delves into a groundbreaking approach to combating microbial threats: the world of antimicrobial nanoparticles. These minuscule entities, engineered at the nanoscale, harness the power of physics and chemistry to interact with microbes in ways previously unimagined. By exploring the intersection of nanotechnology and microbiology, we embark on a journey that promises to redefine how we wage war against infections.

The pages that follow offer a comprehensive exploration of antimicrobial nanoparticles – from their origins and fundamental principles to their cutting-edge applications in medicine, industry, and beyond. We will uncover the science behind their antimicrobial prowess, unravel the mechanisms that grant them their potency, and dissect the intricate dance between nanoparticles and microbes on scales invisible to the naked eye.

The scope of this book extends beyond the laboratory bench, delving into the ethical considerations and societal implications that accompany the emergence of these novel technologies. As we venture into this frontier, questions of safety, regulation, and responsible innovation loom large. How do we balance the extraordinary potential of antimicrobial nanoparticles with the need to ensure their judicious and sustainable use? What challenges must be surmounted to harness their benefits without unintended consequences?

The journey through these pages will introduce you to the pioneers and visionaries who have dedicated their lives to unraveling the secrets of antimicrobial nanoparticles. It will take you through the collaborative efforts of interdisciplinary teams that bridge the gap between nanoscience, medicine, and engineering. It will shed light on the breakthroughs that have already saved lives and transformed industries, while also illuminating the challenges that lie ahead on this uncharted path.

Whether you are a seasoned researcher seeking to expand your horizons, a student eager to explore the cutting edge of science, a healthcare professional grappling with the realities of antimicrobial resistance, or simply a curious mind intrigued by the promises of nanotechnology, this book invites you to join us on a voyage of discovery.

In an age where microbes are ceaselessly evolving, adapting, and challenging our ingenuity, the potential of antimicrobial nanoparticles offers a glimmer of hope. Together, let us embark on this expedition to unlock the potential of these tiny sentinels and forge a new chapter in our ongoing battle for a healthier, safer world.

Welcome to the world of antimicrobial nanoparticles.

Iva Rezić

ACKNOWLEGEMENTS

This book is dedicated to my precious teacher(s) Gyurme Chokyi Sengye Rabjam Rinpoche and Dilgo Khyentse Yangsi Rinpoche, who are an eternal inspiration in becoming a better person, and to my first teachers, mother Renata Penzar and father Josip Penzar, as well as to all mentors and professors I was privileged to work over many years until now.

Many results could have not been discovered without the efforts of multidisciplinary teams and collaboration with dear coworkers from different institutions and universities, so my gratitude goes to all of them.

Last but not least, this book is for you, dear reader, I hope you will find it useful, providing advice, support, and inspiration that will help you in your everyday work.

CHAPTER ONE

NANOREVOLUTION IN MEDICINE[1]

Introduction

Nanoparticles, possessing dimensions spanning 1 to 100 nm, manifest either naturally or through artificial means. They pervade various technological breakthroughs, spanning from intricate electronics to cutting-edge medical treatments. The remarkable strides in nanotechnology have fundamentally transformed the role of nanoparticles, both within the scientific realm and, more recently, across society at large. The realm of medicine has duly acknowledged the significance of polymer-coated nanoparticles, harnessing their exceptional physical, chemical, antibacterial, antimicrobial, and protective attributes. Notably, their biomedical application takes precedence, given that their nanoscale structures align with numerous biological molecules. This alignment bestows them with a myriad of crucial functionalities, encompassing targeted drug conveyance, imaging, photothermal therapy, and sensory applications. Furthermore, adept manipulation at the "nano-scale" level permits the tailoring of their attributes, thus achieving the precise properties requisite for distinct biomedical domains, encompassing electronics, optics, surface plasmon resonance, and physicochemical characteristics.

> Impact of nanotechnology extends deeply into both society and the scientific community. At present, nanomaterials stand at the forefront of advancements in enhancing the functionalities of diverse polymer surfaces, ranging from textiles to items created through 3D printing.

The progress we witness today in the realm of biomedical nanoparticle applications is a direct outcome of the advancements in engineered nanoparticle synthesis and utilization. Within this context, a diverse array of polymeric and metallic nanoparticles is under intense scrutiny for potential biomedical uses. This exploration serves as a pivotal area of

[1] Rezić, I. Nanoparticles for Biomedical Application and Their Synthesis, Polymers 2022, 14, 4961. https://doi.org/10.3390/polym14224961

extensive research, centring on the characterization and refinement of inherent attributes encompassing electronic, optical, and physicochemical traits, alongside the manipulation of surface plasmon resonance. The alteration of specific nanoparticle characteristics, such as size, shape, or aspect ratio, leads to transformative changes in all the aforementioned properties. This process underscores the dynamic nature of nanoparticle modification and its crucial role in shaping their suitability for various biomedical applications. [1]. Nanoparticles exhibit a remarkable capacity for facile synthesis and modification, enabling the induction of unique electronic, optical, magnetic, medical, catalytic, and mechanical attributes. This potent transformation process is responsible for generating a significant surface-to-volume ratio and triggering the quantum size effect, both of which are profoundly influenced by nanoparticle dimensions, configuration, and morphology.

The convergence of nanoparticles and polymers gives rise to materials poised to revolutionize the biomedical landscape. The list of nanoparticles applied on materials for biomedical application is presented in Table 1.1.

Table 1.1. Biomedically applied nanoparticles [1, 2,3].

Nanoparticle	Size	Nanoparticle	Size
Silver, Ag	1.5–350 nm	Magnesium, MgO	20–100 nm
Aluminium, Al	18 or 80 nm	Manganese, Mn_2O_3	30–60 nm
Gold, Au	50–150 nm	Molybdenum, Mo	70 nm
Boron, B_2O_3	40–80 nm	Nickel, Ni	20–50 nm
Barium, $BaSO_4$	1–5 um	Praseodymium, Pr_6O_{11}	15–30 nm
Carbon, C	3–400 nm	Silicon, Si	30–70 nm
Cerium, CeO_2	15–105 nm	Silicon, SiO_2	15–80 nm
Cobalt, Co	28 nm	Samarium, Sm_2O_3	15–55 nm
Chromium, Cr	50 nm	Tin, SnO_2	45–60 nm
Copper, Cu	25–500 nm	Strontium, $SrTiO_3$	100 nm
Dysprosium, Dy_2O_3	30 or 55 nm	Titanium, Ti	30–50 nm
Erbium, Er_2O_3	20–53 nm	Titanium, TiO_2	200 nm
Europium, Eu_2O_3	30–58 nm	Wolfram, W	50 nm
Iron, Fe	25–250 nm	Yttrium, Y_2O_3	20–40 nm
Gadolinium, Gd_2O_3	15–80 nm	Zinc, Zn	80–130 nm
Indium, In_2O_3	30–50 nm	Zinc, Zn	200 nm
Lanthanum, La_2O_3	15–30 nm	Zirconium, ZrC	30–60 nm

Through the strategic incorporation of precise nanoparticles into polymers, a realm of novel materials envisioned as biomedical devices takes shape. These materials find their application in a diverse range of contexts, including woven and nonwoven medical textiles, polymers, and various other practical implementations.

Among the spectrum of diverse engineered nanoparticles, silver nanoparticles are estimated to hold the highest degree of commercialization. [2]. A great diversity of synthetic bottom-up and top-down methods is used for developing and producing nanoparticles of various chemical compositions, sizes, and shapes [3]. Nonetheless, a majority of these techniques rely on wet chemical processes rooted in solution-phase colloidal chemical reactions, frequently entailing rigorous conditions. In addition to these conventional methodologies, nanoparticles can also be synthesized through environmentally friendly approaches that minimize water consumption and operate at lower temperatures. Notably, enzyme-mediated reactions exemplify such green methods that offer a promising alternative for nanoparticle production.

> Production of nanoparticles by green methods efficiently enables industrial application and production in large quantities. Among others, enzymes such are urease or cellulase are very efficient in synthesis of nanoparticles, but have a drawback of being very expensive.

The production of nanoparticles by enzymes offers many advantages: reactions are performed at ambient temperature, moderate pH values are sufficient for an effective enzymatic reactions, the control of reactions is easy, produced nanoparticles can be easily combined with other organic or heat sensitive materials (e.g., proteins), the crystalline phase of the produced nanoparticles can be different from the one(s) obtained by conventional methods and lead to new products, and the morphology of nanoparticles can be controlled by enzymatic reaction engineering.

> Interactions of nanoparticles with living cells are numerous, and currently are under investigation of many multidisciplinary and interdisciplinary researchers. Their toxic effects and influence on the mechanisms of bacteria cells leads to very efficient antimicrobial effects. Such effects are recorded not only on model bacteria systems (gram positive and gram negative) but also against fungi. In addition, the effects were achieved also against microbial strains that are resistant to antibiotics.

A fundamental attribute defining nanoparticles is their scale. Comparisons highlight this significance, as novel engineered nanomaterials match the dimensions of established biological nanostructures. For instance, the DNA double-helix boasts a 2 nm diameter, while the bacteria extend to a length of 200 nm. Nanoparticles encompass precisely this size range. This unique property enables the engineering of colloidal nanoparticles to function as "living nanodrugs," effectively emulating bacteria. Expanding on this concept, the prospect arises for the creation of "robotic nanodrugs." These envisioned entities could be meticulously designed to orchestrate molecular processes within the bodies of humans or animals. Such a paradigm holds the potential to revolutionize medical interventions by precisely manipulating molecular events at the nanoscale. [4].

Interactions of nanoparticles with living organisms

The interaction between nanoparticles and living organisms can be scrutinized across various tiers, spanning from molecular and cellular levels to higher, more systemic tissue levels. This interaction is intricately influenced by diverse routes of administration, encompassing inhalation, intranasal, intravenous, dermal, muscular, and other modalities. This multidimensional interplay engages the exploration of multiple interdisciplinary domains. Researchers from both toxicological and therapeutic perspectives are actively investigating the dynamics of these interactions. Their focus centers on the development of a new breed of nano-immuno-therapeutic drugs, facilitated through comprehensive in vitro and in vivo preclinical trials. However, it's essential to underscore that while the primary interaction of nanoparticles with immune cells hinges on the nanoparticles' physical and chemical characteristics, the mechanisms underlying these interactions remain elusive and cannot be conclusively predicted. [4,5]. Synthetic polymers crafted by human ingenuity undergo meticulous control during their production process, resulting in end products endowed with precisely delineated attributes. These encompass well-defined features such as specific molar mass, distinct architecture, hydrophobic or hydrophilic properties, crystallinity, and strategically positioned functional groups within the molecular structure. Within this context, particular attention is dedicated to gold nanoparticles (Au Nanoparticles), whether unadorned or coated with a polymer layer. This heightened interest stems from the remarkable advantages that position Au nanoparticles as prominent contenders within the diverse realm of nanoparticles tailored for bio-applications.

The pivotal qualities that underscore the prominence of Au nanoparticles are their inherent biocompatibility and the innate simplicity with which their surfaces can be tailored through a wide spectrum of molecules. These attributes bestow upon them a special stature, elevating them to the status of "stars" within the realm of nanoparticles suitable for diverse bio-related applications. (Figure 1.1).

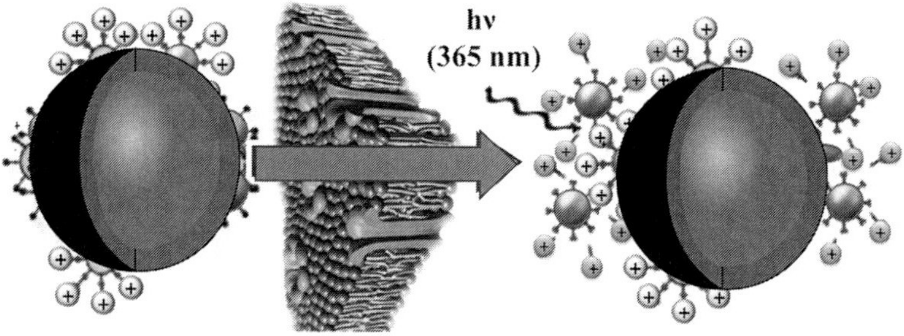

Figure 1.1. Schematic illustration of the photo-induced intracellular controlled release of gold nanospheres. Upon UV irradiation, the photo-labile linker on the gold nanoparticles is cleaved, changing the surface charge of gold nanoparticles from positive to negative and allows the release of the drugs for cancer therapy [5].

The pivotal qualities that underscore the prominence of Au nanoparticles are their inherent biocompatibility and the innate simplicity with which their surfaces can be tailored through a wide spectrum of molecules. These attributes bestow upon them a special stature, elevating them to the status of "stars" within the realm of nanoparticles suitable for diverse bio-related applications. (Figure 1.1). Prominent synthetic methods employed for the production of Au nanoparticles encompass the following techniques: Seed-Mediated Method (Zsigmondy Nuclear Method):

This approach involves a two-step process for generating nano-rods and nano-prisms. It leverages seed particles as a foundation for controlled growth. Thermal Decomposition (Polyol Synthesis): This method utilizes polyvinylpyrrolidone (PVP) as a surface-capping agent. Thermal decomposition within a polyol medium induces nanoparticle formation. Template Mediated Synthesis: Non-spherical Au nanoparticles are crafted in situ, shaped to match a template. Templates can include porous materials' channels, organic surfactants or block polymers, and even biological entities like DNA or viruses. Galvanic Replacement Reaction: Introduced by Brenner and Riddell, this process involves the spontaneous reduction of metal ions into metallic particles and films, operating independently of an external electric field. Distinct from these techniques, enzymatically catalyzed reactions stand out for their environmentally friendly and cost-effective attributes in nanoparticle production.

Within this vast array of controlled synthesis methods, several Au nanoparticle forms hold particular significance due to their yield and reproducibility: Nanorods, Prisms, Shells, Cages: These varied morphologies are meticulously crafted, yielding high-quality nanoparticles with controlled shapes. Hollow Nanostructures (e.g., Stars): These intricate structures boast empty interiors, augmenting their potential applications. Of notable importance are Gold Shells, spherical nanoparticles characterized by a dielectric core (e.g., silica, polystyrene, or sodium sulfide) encased in a thin gold layer. Such techniques and nanoparticle varieties collectively contribute to a diverse toolkit for tailored Au nanoparticle production.

Applications of Au nanoparticles can be categorized into different technological areas (energy, environment, information technologies, and bio-applications) and are based on their outstanding properties [6], such as, for example, optical property to absorb and scatter light with extraordinary efficiency [7] (Genet and Ebbesen, 2007). Recent applications cover the application of Au nanoparticles in photovoltaic devices and environmental conversion of CO into CO_2, as well as in the design of antennas, lenses, and resonators [5]. Important medical applications of Au nanoparticles today are present in drug delivery [8]. Those are proposed for the use of laser irradiation, pH change, ionic concentration change, and similar reactions that trigger a drug release (Figure 1.1).

The exceptional biocompatibility of these nanoparticles renders them amenable to a compelling medical application: their utilization alongside a near-infrared laser source for the controlled thermal ablation of cancerous tissue. This technique holds the promise of minimizing harm to adjacent healthy tissue. Consequently, gold nano shells have made substantial progress and are currently undergoing advanced clinical trials under the scrutiny of the Food and Drug Administration (FDA).

Beyond their role in drug delivery, Au nanoparticles find versatile application within the medical realm. These encompass: Medicine Diagnosis and Therapy: Au nanoparticles play a pivotal role in diagnostics and therapeutic interventions. Their unique properties contribute to precise disease detection and targeted treatments.

Imaging of Tumor Cells: Leveraging the distinctive characteristics of Au nanoparticles, they are employed to facilitate imaging techniques that enhance the visualization of tumor cells.

Additional Diverse Applications: The potential of Au nanoparticles extends to various other medical applications, unlocking innovative approaches in disease management and healthcare.

The multifaceted medical applications of Au nanoparticles underscore their pivotal role in the advancement of medical science and treatment paradigms, as is listed in Table 1.2.

Table 1.2. Imaging and biomedical capabilities of Au nanoparticles [5-10].

Imaging Techniques and Therapy	
Biomedical application	**Nanoparticle morhpology**
Optical scattering	Nano-Au: shells, rods, cages
PET, SPECT	Radioisotope Au^{198}
CT	Au Nanoparticles
Photothermal	Nano-Au: shells, cages
Photoacoustic	NIR-absorbing Au nanoparticles
Chemotherapy	Au nanoparticles loaded with anticancer drugs
Gene therapy	Au nanoparticles loaded with RNA, DNA

There are many methods for characterization of nanoparticles [9]. However, only some of them can reveal the particle size, morphology, and size distribution [2,3]. Among the mostly used methods are scanning electron microscopy (SEM), transmission electron microscopy (TEM), photon correlation spectroscopy (PSC), surface area analysis (BET), and X-ray diffraction (XRF) peak broadening analysis [10]. Characterization methodology is crucial for targeting of special nanoparticles for desired application (Table 1.2). However, specific targeting using desired ligands can be hard to achieve, and the comparison between targeted and non-targeted nanoparticles obtained similar results [4]. Moreover, the interaction of nanoparticles with biological fluids at the contact point site of drug administration (oral, intranasal, or intravenous) makes the problem even more complex. Some strategies are implemented to manipulate this effect, such as PEG nanoparticles that have the ability to avoid interactions with other molecules. Secondly, there are nanoparticles coated with cell membranes that are able to reduce their blood clearance and, thirdly, there are nanoparticles that are able to drain lymph nodes. The array of properties exhibited by nanoparticles profoundly influences their efficacy in reaching their intended targets. Notably, insights garnered from our comprehension of immune system functionality spark innovative concepts for immunotherapeutic applications through alternative administration routes. Examples include intraperitoneal injection or subcutaneous nanoparticle delivery for vaccination purposes. Intriguingly, certain nanoparticle compositions inherently manifest immunostimulatory or immunosuppressive effects, even without the addition of drugs or immune modulators.

Numerous instances substantiate these phenomena, such as hyaluronic acid, PLGA, chitosan nanoparticles, and porous silicon micro particles. These materials have demonstrated the capacity to function as self-adjuvants or elicit M1 or Th1 immune responses.

Nanoparticles offer a plethora of advantages, including their bioactive attributes, seamless integration with other polymeric materials, straightforward composite and bio-composite formation mechanisms, and facile steps for modifying and functionalizing various carriers. However, challenges arise, encompassing strong hydration shells, precipitation-induced turbidity, surface aggregation, dispersive composition, size-related intricacies, and other properties that impede their operational and biomedical applications. Moreover, the diminutive dimensions of nanoparticles give rise to certain drawbacks. Their capacity to readily traverse cell walls, be it in skin or lung cells, raises concerns. Furthermore, their ability to breach the blood-brain barrier adds another layer of potential impact on human health.

In summary, while nanoparticles present remarkable potential for diverse applications, their inherent properties, both advantageous and disadvantageous, necessitate thorough consideration in their deployment for technological and biomedical pursuits.

Polymeric nanoparticles

Certain specialized polymeric nanoparticles are constructed with a central core housing an inner content that could encompass dyes, other inorganic nanoparticles, or drug molecules. Surrounding this core, an outer shell typically consists of hydrophilic polymers. This outer shell can be tailored to incorporate additional functional components, enhancing the nanoparticle's capabilities.

The World Health Organization (WHO) has identified several prevalent chronic diseases afflicting the global human population, including Alzheimer's disease, cardiovascular diseases, cancer, chronic obstructive pulmonary disease, and type 2 diabetes. Chronic inflammation is recognized as a pivotal underlying factor in most chronic diseases. Prolonged immune system activation leads to the production of pro-inflammatory cytokines, causing detrimental effects on organisms. Traditional treatments, involving non-steroidal and anti-inflammatory drugs, lack specificity and often result in various side effects. Furthermore, administering anti-inflammatory drugs presents challenges in achieving optimal bioavailability. Conversely, purposefully designed nanocarriers offer avenues to surmount these hurdles. They allow for targeted drug delivery, addressing specific sites and improving drug solubility. This concept of nano-carrier design is influenced by the inflamed tissue's microenvironment, characterized by heightened permeability, acidic pH, and a significant presence of reactive oxygen species (ROS). These factors contribute to the optimization of treatment outcomes using nanocarriers.

> The World health organization has recognized the problem of antimicrobial resistance as one of the most important problems affecting global human health. Polymeric nanoparticles have a very important role in fighting the most prominent diseases of today human kind.

Nanoparticles in Cancer Treatment

Cancer claims the lives of over 10 million individuals annually, establishing it as the second most common cause of death worldwide. A notable challenge faced by conventional medical treatments is the intricate task of distinguishing between cancerous and healthy cells. However, unique characteristics intrinsic to cancer cells offer novel avenues for targeted approaches. Notably:

Acidic Extracellular Environment: The extracellular milieu of cancer cells tends to be acidic.

Elevated Cell Temperature: Cancer cells often exhibit a higher temperature compared to their surroundings.

Cancer-Associated Enzymes and Surface Molecules: Distinct enzymes and surface molecules are prevalent on cancer cells. These, in conjunction with hypoxic conditions and reactive oxygen species (ROS), define cancerous characteristics.

To address this distinct landscape, polymeric nanoparticles emerge as a versatile solution, amenable to easy modification and manipulation in terms of size and surface properties. Augmenting the effect of passive targeting, these particles are tailored within the size range of 10 to 200 nm, enhancing localization and drug delivery through active targeting mechanisms involving cancer-recognizing molecules.

Diverse polymeric nanoparticle delivery systems for anticancer drugs are under investigation, each targeting specific cancer types. Moreover, curcumin, a natural compound with potential anticancer properties, can be combined with efficient cancer-targeting delivery systems employing biocompatible polymers like PLGA, lecithin, chitosan, silk fibroin, and Eudragit®. Nano-formulated curcumin demonstrates substantial advancements in bioavailability compared to free curcumin, attributing to enhanced adhesion to cancer cells, particularly in the colon.

Incorporating these strategies into the realm of cancer treatment holds promise for improving therapeutic outcomes and enhancing the efficacy of anticancer interventions.

Nanoparticles in Treatment of Infectious Diseases

The escalating resistance of microorganisms to antibiotics poses a grave concern, as underscored by the World Health Organization, which has categorized this issue as a major threat to public health. Within hospital settings, various items with which patients come into contact, such as bedding, towels, sheets, bandages, catheters, and medical equipment, can serve as potential sources of danger if they are not properly sterilized. Consequently, there is an urgent need for technological advancements aimed at producing materials with protective and preventive properties against antibiotic-resistant microorganisms.

Staphylococcus aureus, a bacterium, is capable of causing a range of infections, particularly affecting the skin, soft tissues, bones, and blood vessels. Postoperative surgical procedures frequently result in bloodstream infections, with certain strains even leading to specific symptoms like toxic shock syndrome. The emergence of antibiotic-resistant strains of microorganism's dates back to the 1960s, primarily surfacing within hospital environments. However, over the past decade, the reach of Methicillin-Resistant Staphylococcus Aureus (MRSA) has significantly expanded across multiple countries globally. This proliferation underscores the urgency for preventive measures and novel material development.

Hospitalized individuals with open wounds, those using inhaled devices, and those with compromised immune systems face heightened susceptibility to infections within a broader population. Although MRSA infections post-surgery are relatively uncommon, they may manifest in wounds, the chest, or even the bloodstream, endangering lives and prolonging hospital stays. MRSA infections occur in a range of 1% to 33% of surgical cases, signifying the gravity of the situation and the imperative for effective preventive strategies and materials development.

Addressing the challenge of antibiotic resistance and enhancing infection control within healthcare settings remains a crucial endeavor in safeguarding public health and patient well-being.

Staphylococcus aureus that is resistant to the antibiotics is called the "golden bacteria". It is known to cause severe health problems, such are infections on skin, soft tissues, bones, and blood vessels, which is the most common consequence of postoperative surgery. Some strains of *S. aureus* can cause various specific symptoms including toxic shock syndrome and lead to thousands of deaths all over the world.

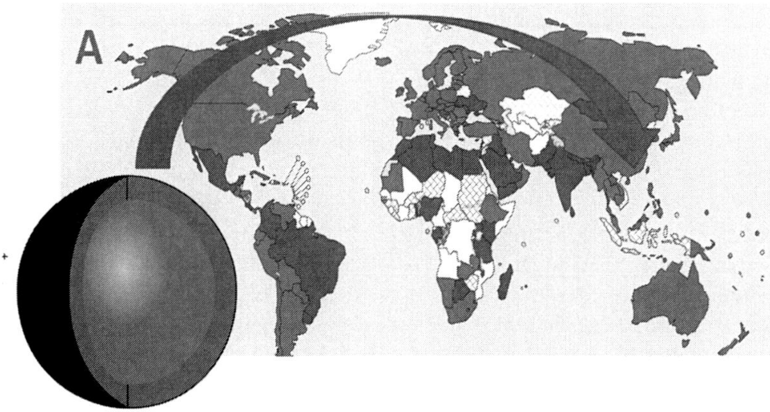

Figure 1.2. (**a**) Graphical illustration of the spread of infections by *S. Aureus* (MRSA), WHO 2014; (**b**) SEM microphotographs of silver nanoparticle;

The initial emergence of penicillin-resistant strains of Staphylococcus aureus (S. aureus) occurred in the mid-1940s. Consequently, S. aureus has been categorized into strains that are either resistant *(MRSA - Methicillin-Resistant Staphylococcus Aureus*) or sensitive (*MSSA - Methicillin-Sensitive Staphylococcus Aureus*) to methicillin. Notably, MRSA infections in hospital settings are associated with a 50% higher likelihood of death compared to MSSA infections. The heightened incidence of MRSA infections within hospitals has prompted increased reliance on alternative antibiotics like vancomycin. However, this elevated usage has contributed to the emergence of vancomycin-resistant S. aureus (VRSA) microorganisms. The evolution of antibiotic-resistant strains continues to pose significant challenges in the realm of healthcare and necessitates vigilant efforts to combat and control their spread. The first such case was described in Japan in 1996 and afterwards in England, France, and the United States [11 -15]. Furthermore, *S. aureus* causes many types of infections: skin (McCaig et al., 2006, [16]); food poisoning (Wieneke et al., 1993 [17]); soft tissues, bones (Sheehy et al., 2010 [18]); blood vessels (Khatib et al., 2009 [19]); endocarditis (Fowler et al., 2005 [20]); or pneumonie [21]. Untreated bacteriemia of *S. aureus* has a mortality rate of 80% [19,22]; most patients do not survive the first year [23] and, in Western European countries, very often patients in hospitals do not receive adequate therapy at the time [22- 26].

A major problem in hospitals is non-sterile materials, because MRSA is easily transmitted through contaminated hands, clothing, or nesterious medical supplies after contact with a patient infected with MRSA either directly (after contact with a patient, blood, tissue fluid, secretions, and excretions) or indirectly (through contaminated instruments, objects, equipment, surfaces, and similar materials). The spread of MRSA can be prevented by the usage of disposable gloves, capes, and masks, but this is not always feasible. Therefore, new materials need to be developed that are active against microorganisms resistant to antibiotics. In the development of new antimicrobial materials, as well as in the functionalization and modification of existing ones, the application of nanoparticles of metal and metal oxides plays a very important role. The nanoparticles have excellent new medical, mechanical, optical, magnetic, catalytic, and electronic properties owing to a specific surface that is highly dependent on their size, structure, and shape. The global demand for nanoparticles of metal and metal oxide is projected to grow to 1700 tons in 2020 [5].

Nanoparticles have strong antibacterial activity on a wide range of Gram-positive and Gram-negative bacteria, including strains resistant to antibiotics [24]. They have great application because of their chemical stability, catalytic activity, and high conductivity. Rezić et al. have shown that silver nanoparticles have higher antibacterial activity owing to their high surface-to-volume ratio, which ensures better contact with microorganisms [4]. Furthermore, Al-Dhabi et al. have demonstrated visible antimicrobial activity against pathogenic wound infections such as *Bacillus subtilis, Enterococcus faecalis, Staphylococcus epidermidis,* multidrug-resistant *Staphylococcus aureus,* and *Escherichia coli* [25]. Silver nanoparticles with their own antimicrobial activity in combination with antibiotics (such as penicillin G, amoxicillin, erythromycin, clindamycin, or vancomycin) enhance the action of antibiotics in the treatment of resistant *Staphylococcus aureus* and *Escherichia coli* infections [26]. The interaction between nanoparticles and microorganisms is complex. Two interrelated mechanisms are described in the literature: (1) membrane potential disturbance and (2) production of reactive oxygen species (ROS), where nano-particles act as nano-catalysts [27,28]. Microbial membrane damage occurs when nanoparticles electrostatically bind to the surface of the bacterium, resulting in changes in the membrane wall and membrane potential and loss of integrity. Reactive oxygen species (ROS) are the cytotoxicity of nanoparticles in vivo and in vitro conditions where oxidative stress on the surface damages the integrity of microbial membranes by lipid peroxidation, further damaging the protein and enzyme function and damaging DNA and RNA. In some cases, ROS is induced by either visible or UV light and photocatalytic nanoparticle toxicity, such as, for example, TiO_2 nanoparticles, which, under UV light, cause lipid peroxidation, respiratory dysfunction, and death of methicillin-resistant *Staphylococcus aureus* cells [29]. Other mechanisms of toxicity of bacterial cell nanoparticles include direct inhibition of specific essential enzymes, induction of nitrogen reactive species [30], and induction of programmed cell death or apoptosis [31]. Table 1.3 shows the activity of silver nanoparticles of various dimensions on microorganisms.

Table 1.3. Antimicrobial activity of silver nanoparticles on microorganisms [3,9,32].

Silver Nanoparticles size, nm	Activity	Microorganisms
5–30	Antibacterial	*Acinetobacter baumannii*
~20–100	Growth inhibition	*Acinetobacter*
~20–100	Growth inhibition	*Aeromonas*
104.9	Antifungal	*Aspergillus foetidus*
5–30	Antifungal	*Aspergillus fumigatus*
4.75–8.31	Antifungal	*Aspergillus niger*
104.9	Antifungal	*Aspergillus oryzae*
7–20	Antifungal	*Aspergillus*
Not specified	Antifungal	*Aspergillus terreus*
120	Antibacterial	*Bacillus cereus*
24	Antibacterial	*Bacillus megaterium*
16	Bactericide	*Bacillus mycoides*
Not specified	Bactericide	*Bacillus pumulis*
~100	Antibacterial	*Bifidobacterium*
~20–~30	Growth inhibition	*Bordetella pertussis*
~20–45	Antifungal	*Candida albicans*
Not specified	Antifungal	*Candida glabrata ATCC90030*
Not specified	Antifungal	*Candida tropicalis*
~20–100	Growth inhibition	*Citrobacter*
50–70	Antifungal	*Cryptococcus neoformans*
8–12	Bactericide	*Eschericia coli MTCC 443*
8–12	Antibacterial	*Enterobacter aerogenes*
~89	Antibacterial	*Enterococcus faecalis*
104.9	Antifungal	*Fusarium oxysporum*
~6	Antibacterial	*Klebsiella pneumoniae*
16	Bactericide	*Lactobacillus acidophilus*
17–29	Antibacterial	*Listeria monocytogenes*
198–595	Growth inhibition	*MRSA*
~20–~30	Growth inhibition	*Micrococcus luteus*

20–30	Inhibition of biofilm formation	*multidrug resistant Pseudomonas aeruginosa*
~6	Antibacterial	*Multidrug Resistant Escherichia coli*
~6	Antibacterial	*Multidrug Resistant Klebsiella pneumoniae*

Table 1.3 continues. Antimicrobial activity of silver nanoparticles [3,9,32].

Silver Nanoparticles size, nm	Activity	Microorganisms
~10–~100	Bactericide	*Staphylococcus aureus*
~10	Antibacterial	*Paenibacillus koreensis*
>42	Antifungal	*Penicillium*
~100	Antibacterial	*Peptostreptococcus*
9–10	Antifungal	*Pichia pastoris*
20–70	Antibacterial	*Propionibacterium acnes*
Not specified	Cytotoxic	*Proteus mirabilis*
50–70	Antibacterial	*Proteus vulgaricus*
1–12	Antibacterial	*Pseudomonas aeruginosa*
~2–40	Antifungal	*Rhizoctonia bataticola*
~15	Antifungal	*Saccharomyces*
63–90	Antibacterial	*Salmonella paratyphi*
Not specified	Antifungal	*Scedosporium JAS1*
Not specified	Antibacterial	*Serratia marcescens*
17–29	Antibacterial	*Shigella flexneri MTCC 1475*
1–12	Antibacterial	*Staphylococcus aureus*
5–25	Antibacterial	*Staphylococcus aureus 25923*
~89	Antibacterial	*Staphylococcus aureus BAA-1721*
20–70	Antibacterial	*Staphylococcus epidermidis*
15	Antibacterial	*Streptococcus*
~15	Antifungal	*Trichopyton rubrum*
5–25	Antibacterial	*Vibrio cholerae*
~54	Antibacterial	*Xanthomonas campestris*
Not specified	Antibacterial	*Yersinia enterocolitica*

Polymers containing metal nanoparticles and metal oxides have antimicrobial effects [32], but their effects on many pathogenic microorganisms have not yet been sufficiently explored.

As can be seen from the table 1.3. in the effects against different strains of the same bacteria, not only the chemical composition of the nanoparticles plays a significant role (since all nanoparticles presented in Table 1.3. are silver nanoparticles), but the efficiency strongly depends on the size of the particular nanomaterial.

Antibiotics usually target bacterial cell membrane synthesis, translation, and DNA replication [33]. The resistance to antibiotics can occur on each of these antimicrobial effects.

The primary mechanism through which nanoparticles exert their effects involves direct interaction with the bacterial membrane. This process does not necessarily entail membrane penetration or breaching the cell wall. This unique mode of action provides microorganisms with less opportunity to develop resistance against nanoparticles. Currently, silver nanoparticles find application in various coatings, such as those used on surgical instruments, catheters, masks, orthopaedic implants, and dental materials. They are incorporated into these materials to enhance their properties. Additionally, silver nanoparticles contribute to diagnostics by increasing the sensitivity of bio-detection techniques. These nanoparticles are employed in highly sensitive clinical tests, ranging from diagnosing myocardial infarction to fluorescence-based detection of RNA. The versatile applications of silver nanoparticles underscore their potential to advance diverse fields, from healthcare to diagnostics and beyond. [34] (Table 1.4).

Table 1.4. Application of silver nanoparticles in medicine items [35].

Treatment	Effect of Silver Nanoparticles
Anaesthesiology	Coating on breathing masks, endotracheal tubes for mechanical ventilation assistance
Cardiology	Coating on the tracking catheter
Stomatology	Adhesives in dental materials, silver-filled SiO_2 nanocomposite resins
Diagnostics	Ultra-sensitive and ultra-fast platform for clinical tests for myocardial infarction diagnosis, fluorescence detection of RNA
Drug release	Remote laser induced opening microcapsules
Eye care	Contrasts on contact lenses
Visualisation	Nomenclatures for marking cells
Neurosurgery	Coating of the catheter for the drainage of cerebrospinal fluid
Orthopaedics	Bone cement additives, joint replacement implants, orthopaedic socks
Drugs	Treatments for dermatitis, ulcerative colitis and acne, HIV-1 inhibition

Surgery	Coats in medical textiles—surgical suits and masks
Urology	Plastered on surgical nets for pelvic reconstruction

In addition to the pharmaceutical industry, nanoparticles of silver are used in the cosmetic industry thanks to their strong antibacterial and anti-inflammatory properties, in cosmetic products such as deodorants, anti-aging creams, and so on. Nanotechnology can solve the problem of bio-film formation by using an antibacterial active surface with a combination of ZnO and MgO nanoparticles that is activated in the dark and is effective against *MRSA* species [36].

Considering the new solutions, it is not surprising that resistance to nanoparticles by microorganisms has already occurred; Panaček et al. demonstrated that gram-negative bacteria *of Escherichia coli 013, Pseudomonas aeruginosa CCM 3955* and *E. coli CCM 3954* can develop resistance to silver nanoparticles after repeated exposure and resistance results from the production of adhesive flagellin protein, which activates the aggregation of nanoparticles [37]. Research into antimicrobial nanoparticle coatings has found intriguing applications in the realm of space exploration. Notably, the International Space Station (ISS) has conducted experiments with coatings composed of silver and ruthenium. These coatings exhibited remarkable efficacy against both Gram-negative and Gram-positive bacterial strains, including highly resistant pathogenic bacteria such as *MRSA, Enterococcus faecalis, Staphylococcus epidermidis, E. coli, Pseudomonas aeruginosa, Acinetobacter baumannii*, and *Legionella.* The ISS, characterized by its confined and isolated environment, presents unique challenges in terms of bacterial growth. In this environment, bacteria can evolve specialized antibiotic defence mechanisms, such as developing thicker cell walls or upregulating virulent genes. Furthermore, microgravity and cosmic radiation can contribute to enhancing the virulence of microorganisms, potentially transforming them into more potent pathogens. The distinct conditions within the ISS, coupled with reduced immune defences among astronauts due to microgravity and cosmic radiation, create an environment that is particularly conducive to infections. This susceptibility is further exacerbated by the psychological stress associated with space travel. As a result, astronauts become more vulnerable to infections, necessitating innovative approaches such as antimicrobial nanoparticle coatings to mitigate the risks posed by various microorganisms in the unique space environment. [38].

Nanoparticles in Implants and Prosthetics

Nanoparticles find extensive application in the realm of implantable devices, where specific attributes are essential. Implantable devices necessitate qualities such as excellent biocompatibility, tissue compatibility, resistance to corrosion, and notably, antibacterial properties. A diverse array of classical medical devices, implants, and prosthetics encompass this category, including catheters, dental implants, pacemakers, prostheses, and more. These materials engage in prolonged, direct contact with biological tissues, making their biocompatibility a pivotal consideration that governs their usability.

Problems frequently encountered with implantable devices are linked to their biocompatibility, giving rise to issues such as toxicity, allergic reactions, inflammation, and, at times, bacterial infections. The integration of nanoparticles in the design and fabrication of these devices offers a multifaceted approach to address these challenges. By bestowing antibacterial properties, nanoparticles enhance the safety and effectiveness of implantable devices, effectively mitigating the risks associated with microbial infections. The utilization of nanoparticles in the creation of implantable devices marks a significant advancement in biomedical engineering, poised to revolutionize the field by improving the longevity, functionality, and overall compatibility of these critical medical tools [39].

Nanoparticles as Theragnostic Devices

Therapeutic systems exhibit a dual role, serving both as a therapeutic and diagnostic agent. These systems are meticulously engineered to achieve target-specific drug delivery while concurrently monitoring the drug release process. Furthermore, they possess the capability to track the progression of disease and the response to treatment. In contrast to traditional diagnostic imaging techniques employing inorganic contrast agents for methods like magnetic resonance imaging, computed tomography, and angiography, organic fluorophores emerge as a promising alternative due to their favorable safety profile.

These systems find diverse applications, extending to formulations for skin, hair, nails, and various other contexts. For specific applications, nanoparticles of varying sizes (ranging from 50 to 500 nm) are employed, capitalizing on their ability to penetrate the skin and reach deeper layers within the organism. This attribute has facilitated the development of "transdermal drugs," wherein therapeutic agents are administered through the skin, enabling efficient and controlled delivery of treatments.

By merging therapeutic and diagnostic functionalities, these innovative systems pave the way for more precise and personalized medical interventions, advancing the frontiers of both diagnosis and treatment in the field of healthcare [39]. Polymers used as carriers are chitosan, albumin, PLGA, or PLA. In addition, inorganic nanoparticles are useful in antibacterial coating; thus, for example, TiO_2 coated with silver-doped hydroxyapatite or silver-coated collagen proved to possess antibacterial activity useful for catheters and dental implants effective against *S. aureus* and *P. aeruginosa* [40].

Nanoparticles Synthesis by Enzymes

The first attempt of synthesis of metallic particles by enzymes was performed by McConnel and Frajola (1961), when the synthesis of carbonate apatite was carried out in the presence of carbon anhydrase. Today, the advents and developments in nanotechnology resulted in a wide range of microorganisms and their enzymes, which can be utilized in the production of nanoparticles. Some examples of synthesis of biomedically applicable nanoparticles are presented in Table 1.5

Table 1.5. Nanoparticles synthesized by microorganisms [41–44].

Microorganisms	Nanoparticle	Temperature, °C	Size (nm)	Shape
Rhodococcus species	Au	37	5–15	sphere
Shewanella oneidensis	Au	30	12 ± 5	sphere
Plectonemaboryanum	Au	25–100	<10–25	cube
Plectonema boryanum	Au	25	10–600	octahedral
Escherichia coli	Au	37	20–30	triangle
Yarrowia lipolytica	Au	30	15	triangle
Rhodopseudomonas capsulate	Au	30	10–20	sphere
Brevibacterium casei	Au, Ag	37	10–50	sphere
Trichoderma viride	Ag	27	5–40	sphere
Phaenerochaete chrysosporium	Ag	37	50–200	pyramidal
Bacillus cereus	Ag	37	4–5	sphere
Lactobacillus species	Ba, TiO_3	25	20–80	tetragonal
Fusarium oxysporum	CdSe	10	9–15	sphere
Escherichia coli	Cd,Te	37	2.0–3.2	sphere
Fusariumoxysporum	$CdCO_3$, $PbCO_3$	27	120–200	sphere

Lactobacillus	CdS	25–60	4.9 ± 0.2	sphere
Pyrobaculum islandicum	Cr, Mn, U, Tc	100	different	sphere
Shewanella oneidensis	Fe_3O_4	28	40–50	hexagonal
Enterobacter species	Hg	30	2–5	sphere
Desulfovibrio desulfuricans	Pd	25	50	sphere
Shewanella algae	Pt	25	5	-
Saccharomyces cerevisiae	Sb_2O_3	25–60	2–10	sphere
Shewanella species	Se	30	181 ± 40	sphere
Fusarium oxysporum	$SrCO_3$	27	10–50	needle like
Fusarium oxysporum	TiO_2	300	6–13	sphere
Fusarium oxysporum	ZrO_2	25	3–11	sphere

Nanoparticle synthesis involves three main chemical pathways: the Turkevich method, Brust–Schiffrin method, and seed growth method. John Turkevich introduced his method in 1951, utilizing sodium citrate as both a reducing agent and stabilizer to produce spherical nanoparticles ranging from 10 to 20 nm in size. The Brust–Schiffrin method, established in 1994, facilitates the creation of nanoparticles sized between 1.5 and 5.2 nm through the use of thiole under ambient conditions. The seed growth method provides precise control over nanoparticle size and shape, contributing to its efficacy.

In contrast to conventional chemical synthetic routes, green methods have emerged as sustainable alternatives, employing plant extracts or microorganisms to synthesize nanoparticles. These green approaches aim to reduce reliance on toxic chemicals traditionally used in nanoparticle synthesis. By utilizing herbal extracts, the reduction step within this process still qualifies it as a green synthesis method. An added advantage of this approach is that nanoparticles produced using this methodology often do not necessitate further functionalization agents.

Numerous biopolymers play a role in nanoparticle synthesis through green methods. These include PVP (polyvinylpyrrolidone), PEG (polyethylene glycol), polyvinyl alcohol, polyacrylamide, polyallylamine, polyphenols, and polymethyl aminoethyl methacrylate. Additionally, various surfactants can be employed to facilitate these reactions. The adoption of green synthesis not only aligns with sustainable practices but also offers a more benign and environmentally friendly route to obtaining nanoparticles with potential applications in various fields. [39].

The nanoparticles can also be prepared using biopolymers. Such a procedure can be performed using a single biopolymer or their combination with other reducing agents. Some of the useful biopolymers are as follows: pectin, glucose, dextrin, amino-dextrin, gum Arabic, starch, chitosan, proteins, gelatin, collagen, casein, tyrosine, alpha-amylase, aspartic acid, tyrosine, tryptophan, glutamic acid, sodium glutamate, cystine, and L-leucine, among others [39.] The organic reagents used are as follows: amino alcohols, glycerol, luminol, nitriloacetic acid, and sodium rhodizonate, enabling the reduction of gold nanoparticles from $HAuCl_4$.

Enzymatic synthesis of nanoparticles at moderate temperatures will be investigated in this chapter, because it is of prime interest for the industry; that is, mild manufacturing conditions will ensure low energy consumption, economical production, less manpower, and compatibility with other fabrication processes.

Nanoparticles can be effectively utilized in medical applications, especially for cancer treatment, when combined with proteins. The integration of nanoparticles with proteins opens up avenues for therapies that target cancer cells precisely. Furthermore, when nanoparticles are synthesized using enzyme-mediated reactions, the resulting chemical and physical properties of the nanoparticles can differ from those produced through conventional methods. This diversity in properties offers a range of novel applications for these nanoparticles.

By comprehending this mechanism, reactions can be guided to produce nanoparticles with specific properties suited for various applications. Enzymes, functioning as protein catalysts, exhibit a high degree of specificity for their substrates. They drive specific chemical reactions such as hydrolysis, reduction-oxidation, phase transition, elimination of specific functional groups, and isomerization. While enzymatic reactions naturally occur within living organisms, technological advancements have enabled their utilization in bioreactors within scientific and industrial laboratories. This capability allows for the production of diverse chemical compounds, including drugs and detergent products, as well as nanoparticles.

The incorporation of enzymes into nanoparticle synthesis processes not only expands the scope of potential applications but also aligns with sustainable and targeted therapeutic strategies. This interdisciplinary approach capitalizes on the inherent properties of both enzymes and nanoparticles to develop innovative solutions for medical and industrial challenges. [45].

Urease is a very interesting enzyme for producing nanoparticles. It can be isolated from different microorganisms (*Aspergillus niger, Proteus mirabilis, Bacillus subtilis,* and *Aerobacter aerogenes)* and applied for the production of nanoparticles of different morphologies like thin films, hollow micro- and nano-spheres, nanotubes, 2D patterns, 3D replicas of biominerals, and others [43]. Therefore, the *urease*-mediated synthesis of nanoparticles is an attractive research field that enables the possibilities of producing nanoparticles for a wide variety of applications: in cancer therapy, for producing materials of special purposes, in food packing, geotextiles, and many others [46].

Methods for producing nanoparticles by *urease*-catalysed reactions can be divided into two main categories: (i) reactions in which the precipitants of metal ions are produced by enzymatic reactions (metal ions in solutions precipitate into oxides, hydroxides, carbonates, or phosphates), and (ii) reactions in which enzymes directly interact with metal-containing substrates to produce metallic materials [42].

Reactions using *urease* are usually very simple and obtained nanoparticles can be formed as hydroxides, carbonates, hydratized oxides, or other chemical species. For example, if a small amount of *urease* is diluted in a solution containing calcium chloride and urea, the *urease* will hydrolyze urea into ammonia (carbonic acid will also be produced). In the same reaction, calcium ions react with the carbonate at room temperature, and calcium carbonate is produced [47,48]:

$$H_2NCONH_2 + 2\ H_2O \rightarrow 2\ NH_3 + H_2CO_3$$

$$Ca^{2+} + CO_3^{2-} \rightarrow CaCO_3$$

The crystallinity, size, and mechanism of growth of produced nanoparticles are governed by reaction parameters (e.g., concentrations, stirring, pH, temperature, pressure, and ultrasound effects). In this project, the kinetic of such enzymatically catalyzed reactions will be thoroughly investigated by different classical instrumental methods. In addition, *beyond-state-of-the-art* analytical and bioanalytical methods will be implemented for revealing the mechanisms of preselected reactions. Unuma et al. (2004) applied *urease* immobilized on alginate gel particles to produce porous aluminum nanoparticles [43]. In this reaction, after reaction (1), the following reaction occurred:

$$Al^{3+} + 3NH_3 + 3H_2O \rightarrow Al(OH)_3 + 3\ NH_4^+$$

Under high temperatures, aluminum hydroxide produced in reaction (3) converts into Al_2O_3 with a particle size of 1–2 mm (Unuma et al., 2004). Porous nanoparticles of iron oxide are produced by a similar reaction:

$$Fe^{3+} + xOH^- + nH_2O \rightarrow FeO_{y/2}(OH)_{3-y} \times mH_2O$$

In contrast to the process of producing aluminum nanoparticles (reaction 3), process (4) also utilizes the polymer matrices molecules, which degrade after drying and calcification in order to obtain porous iron NP structures [49]. In the reaction of *urease* with ammonia and carbonates, many other metallic nanoparticles can be produced: magnetite [50], iron hydroxide [51], aluminum sulfate [52], calcium carbonate [47,53], strontium and barium carbonate [48], calcium phosphate [54], yttrium hydroxide [55], magnesium oxide, and zinc oxide, in the form of nano-shells (Figure 1.3).

Targeted products' metallic nanoparticles have biological and medical activity, antimicrobial, water-repellent, and other protective and polymer-applicable properties. Owing to the special characteristics of the mechanism of its reaction, catalytic *urease* processes can be used for the synthesis of Al, Au, Ca, Cr, Fe, Ge, Pd, Pt, Ti, Y, Zn, and Zr nanoparticles. Some of those Nanoparticles (Ca, Ge, Pd, and Pt) are currently not applied in medical materials, while others (Zn and Zr) are applied only as oxides (Table 1.1). The produced nanoparticles are subsequently deposited onto a polymer substrate in the form of a thin film. The application of such a coated protective material is foreseen for medical applications. *Urease* is not the only enzyme that can be used. In addition, four oxidoreductases can be utilized: *cellobiose dehydrogenase* (CDH), *glucose dehydrogenase, glucose oxidase*, and *laccase*. These enzymes have many applications in biotechnology and are used for producing metallic nanoparticles. For example, *glucose oxidase* extracted from *Aspergillus niger* can be used for production of different nanoparticles (e.g., Au, Sn, and others) [53].

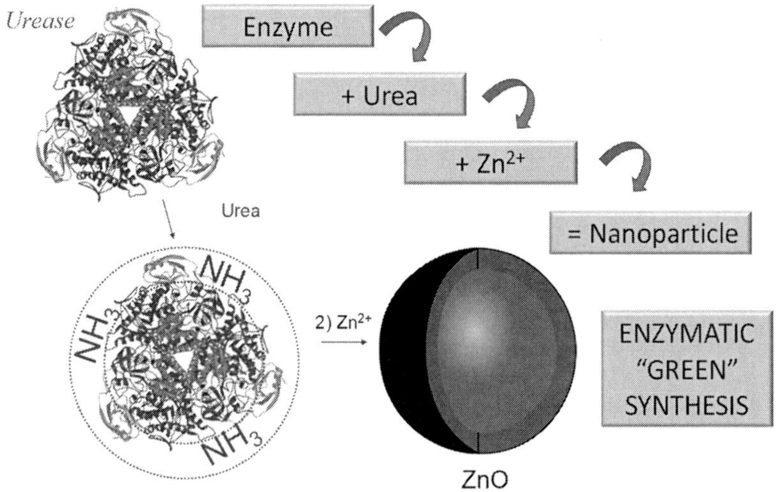

Figure 1.3. Synthesis of ZnO nano shells using the *urease* enzyme as a catalytic template. In the first step, NH_3 is generated by the hydrolysis of urea. This adjusts the pH value around the enzyme. In the second step, Zn^{2+} is added. The growth of nano shells is governed by the local pH value at the enzyme/solution interface (De la Rica and Matsui, 2008).[1].

Enzymatic synthesis of nanoparticles is not the only green approach available today, but it offers so many advantages that many researchers are developing new methods and new sources of enzymes in order to enhance their efficiency. In addition, by genetic modelling the new sources of enzymes are modified and produced enabling even greater possibility of new applications.

Application of CDH enzyme for producing gold nanoparticles is reported in the literature [54]. Their results show that CDH acts as an electron donor and reduces gold from $[AuCl_4]^-$ complex into metallic gold nanoparticle by direct electron transfer (DET) at pH 5 or by mediated electron transfer (MET) at pH 7. The limiting factor for nanoparticles' growth is the ability of CDH to interact with the growing Au nanoparticles.

This is an important fact, useful for controlling the direction of the reaction. For example, the ability of enzymes to control the rate of nucleation of nanoparticles is the key step in using them as plasmatic nano-sensors. Having all of this in mind, Au nanoparticles should be the first targeted metal ion for biomedical applications [56, 57].

There are many different methods for revealing the mechanisms of metallic nanoparticles' biomedical application: *"beyond-state-of-the-art"* instrumental methods such as gas-phase electrophoretic mobility molecular analyzer (GEMMA) [58–61], parallel differential mobility analyzer (PDMA) [62], and liquid chromatography/capillary electrophoresis coupled to MALDI and ESI mass spectrometry (LC/CE-MS/MS), as well as classical spectroscopic methods (graphite furnace atomic absorption spectrometry (GF-AAS), inductively coupled plasma optical emission spectrometry (ICP-OES) [63–66], scanning electron microscopy equipped with the EDX detector (SEM-EDX) [67,68], thermal gravimetric analysis (TGA), Fourier transform infrared spectroscopy (FTIR), UV/VIS spectroscopy, and liquid chromatography (HPLC)), which is convenient to provide important information on mechanisms of reactions and obtaining products of desired crystallinity, size, and shape [69–72]. The identification of the newly isolated enzymes can be performed by MALDI-TOF/TOF-MS and LC-MS/MS methods.

Special focus and attention should be given to the determination of the kinetics of the systems studied, as well as to the revealing of the mechanisms of reaction by *"beyond-state-of-the-art-techniques"* GEMMA and PDMA coupled to capillary electrophoresis (CE), which were invented and developed by prof. Allmaier et al., for the analysis of nanosize materials.

To the best of our knowledge, the application of GEMMA and PDMA to monitor enzymatic in situ reactions and to follow both of the enzymes and produce nanoparticles, i.e., the size-separated nanoparticles are collected and can be investigated by other techniques as SEM or AFM, is a new, beyond-state-of-the-art concept in the field.

Although different *state-of-the-art* techniques can be today utilized for the in situ measurement of nanoparticles [73–77], such attempts cannot provide insight into the particle growth. In future work, on the other hand, the focus should be shifted to understanding the mechanism of nanoparticles' growth during the reaction by monitoring reactants and products (enzymes and occurred metallic nanoparticles). Having the possibility to obtain a deep insight into the mechanism of enzymatically guided reactions is crucial, as contradictory observations and conclusions are currently reported in highly ranked scientific journals (*Nature* and *Angewandte Chemie*). For example, B. Sharma et al. (2013) concluded that, during *urease*-guided reaction of the formation of hollow ZnO nanoparticles, the enzyme covers the outer shell (Sherma et al., 2013). This conclusion is in contradiction to the interpretation of De la Rica and Matsui (2008), who reported that the enzyme (Figure 3) fulfills the nanoparticles' inner core [78].

Widely used nanoparticles include oxides of Al, Sb, Bi, Ce, Cu, In/Sn, Fe, Mg, Mn, Ni, Si, Ti, Y, Zn, and Zr, thanks to their novel electronic, optical, magnetic, medical, catalytic, and mechanical properties resulting from the high surface-to-volume ratio and quantum size effect. The primary target of biomedical application research should be to modify and control protective materials using newly prepared nanoparticles (e.g., Ag, Al, Au, Cr, Ge, Fe, Pd, Pt, Ti, Y, Zn, and Zr nanoparticles). Polymer materials coated with thin films of nanoparticles have special protective properties, such as preventing oxygen, moisture, and microorganism permeability. The process of thin film deposition is very important, as it influences graininess and the structure of the deposit. In other words, the deposit can comprise grains of different sizes and its structure may suffer from defects in connectivity [79].

There are several thin film deposition technologies that can be applied: sputtering, sol–gel deposition, spray coating, chemical vapor deposition, spray pyrolysis, cathode electro deposition, anodic conversion, and conventional evaporation. The properties of thin metal films with nano-holes smaller than the light wavelength have recently attracted large amounts of interest, owing to the remarkable observation of extraordinary light transmission through metallic sub-wavelength hole arrays, which does not obey classical optical theory [80]. Therefore, several methodologies should be tested including the sol–gel process of dip coating [81–84]. Such methodologies are very useful in combining different nanoparticles and different polymer materials [85,86], in order to create metal nanoparticle films of different thicknesses that are the most efficient for biomedical applications (Figure 1. 4) [87].

Characterization of nanoparticles

The important nanoparticles in biomedical applications are inorganic and organic nanoparticles. Among inorganic species, gold nanoparticles and silver nanoparticles are today the most investigated and prominent species.

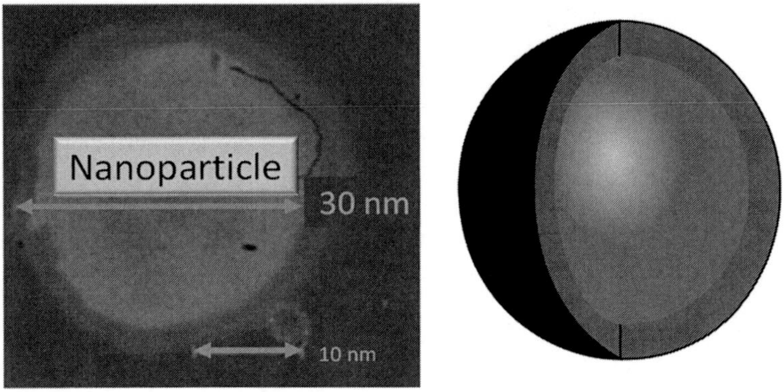

Figure 1.4. SEM magnified image of gold Nanoparticle obtained by *cellobiose dehydrogenase* treatment of $[AuCl_4]^-$ (Malel et al., 2010) and its graphical presentation.

The benefits of nanoparticles in biomedical applications, along with their synthesis methods, have been extensively discussed in this study. However, it is crucial to acknowledge that these nanomaterials can also possess significant toxicity. The extent of their toxicity hinges on various factors, including their physical, chemical, and morphological properties. Prior to selecting the optimal synthesis pathway for nanoparticle production, careful consideration of their potential toxic effects is imperative. Through strategic optimization of the synthesis process, key parameters like size, shape, composition, and other vital characteristics should be systematically manipulated to ensure that the resultant nanoparticles do not induce adverse toxic responses.

By conscientiously engineering nanoparticles to achieve desired properties, it becomes possible to minimize or entirely circumvent their inherent toxicity. For instance, factors such as size, surface area, shape, aspect ratio, surface coating, crystalline structure, dissolution rate, and agglomeration play pivotal roles. These factors collectively influence the nanoparticles' capacity to generate reactive species (ROS) and engage in other mechanisms that contribute to cytotoxicity, genotoxicity, and neurotoxicity processes.

Strategically navigating the synthesis process with a comprehensive understanding of the interplay between nanoparticle properties and potential toxic effects allows for the development of safer nanomaterials with minimal risk in biomedical applications. This approach aligns with responsible and ethical nanotechnology practices, ensuring the advancement of innovative therapies and technologies without compromising safety.

Several toxic mechanisms have been identified in the context of nanoparticles, encompassing the induction of reactive species formation, cytotoxicity to cells, and genotoxic and neurotoxic effects. Notably, smaller nanoparticles tend to exhibit a higher rate of acute toxicity in in vivo experiments. In contrast to this field, the realm of polymeric nano-sized materials offers a much broader scope, facilitating the development of a wide range of targeting materials with diverse applications.

Nanomaterials hold immense promise in technological and industrial domains, with several intriguing future prospects. Carbon nanotubes, characterized by their unique physical properties, have the potential to revolutionize automobile design by enabling electrical and thermal conductivity. Additionally, the realm of nano-robots is on the horizon, representing the next stage in miniaturization. These nano-robots could assist the cells of living organisms in their daily tasks, offering an innovative approach to various applications.

Furthermore, the concept of nano and micro vehicles capable of movement and guidance on specific surfaces has garnered attention. This technology has implications across numerous aspects of life, offering opportunities for enhanced functionality and efficiency.

The rapid growth of nanomaterial science is leading to the integration of nanoparticles into various innovative applications across industries. This evolution is poised to bring about groundbreaking advancements that have the potential to reshape multiple sectors and profoundly influence human life.

The combination of biomedically active nanoparticles with different polymers, whether in the form of thin films, nano capsules, or other configurations, holds the promise of yielding new materials with altered physical, chemical, and mechanical properties. These materials could exhibit traits such as antimicrobial activity, water repellence, and low oxygen permeability, which are advantageous for biomedical surfaces.

Hollow nanoparticles designed to release encapsulated molecules could be employed in targeted drug delivery systems. Furthermore, polymers coated with nanoparticles offer potential benefits for applications like catheters and prosthetic materials.

In contrast to many existing review articles that focus on a single type of nanoparticle, this manuscript provides a comprehensive exploration of various nanoparticles, including both inorganic (silver, gold) and organic (polymeric) species. A distinctive aspect of this work lies in its coverage not only of potential biomedical applications but also the toxicological implications of nanoparticles. By strategically influencing synthesis parameters, the mitigation of toxicity can be achieved, underscoring the importance of an integrated approach to crafting desirable nanomaterials for real-world applications.

The practical application of these newly developed biomedically active materials hinges on their toxicity, environmental impact, and production costs. As interdisciplinary researchers collaborate and share knowledge, significant strides are expected in addressing specific challenges within analytical chemistry, material sciences, and nanotechnology concerning biomedically active nanoparticles.

The trajectory of nanomaterial research is set to foster an era of innovation, with the potential to revolutionize industries, improve human health, and usher in a new paradigm of technological possibilities.

References

1. Khursheed, R.; Dua, K.; Vishwas, S.; Gulati, M.; Jha, N.K.; Aldhafeeri, G.M.; Alanazi, F.G.; Goh, B.H.; Gupta, G.; Paudel, K.R.; et al. Biomedical applications of metallic nanoparticles in cancer: Current status and future perspectives. *Biomed. Pharmacother.* **2022**, *150*, 112951.
2. Rezić, I. Determination of engineered nanoparticles on textiles and in textile wastewaters. *TrAC Trends Anal. Chem.* **2011**, *30*, 1159–1167.
3. Rezić, I. Engineered Nanoparticles in Textiles Textile Wastewaters. In *Analysis Risk of Nanomaterials in Environmental Food Samples*; COAC, Farre, M., Barcelo, D., Eds.; Elsevier: Chennai, India, 2012; Volume 59, pp. 235–264.
4. Anfray, C.; Mainini, F.; Andón, F.T. Nanoparticles for immunotherapy. *Front. Nanosci.* **2020**, *16*, 265–306.
5. Jesus, M.D.L.F.; Grazu, V. *Nanobiotechnology: Inorganic Nanoparticles vs Organic Nanoparticles, Frontiers of Nanoscience*; Palmer, R.E., Ed.; Elsevier: Oxford, UK, 2012; Volume 4.
6. Lopez-Sanchez, J.A.; Dimitratos, N.; Hammond, C.; Brett, G.L.; Kesavan, L.; White, S.; Miedziak, P.; Tiruvalam, R.; Jenkins, R.L.; Carley, A.F.; et al. Facile removal of stabilizer-ligands from supported gold nanoparticles. *Nat. Chem.* **2011**, *3*, 551–556.
7. Genet, C.; Ebbesen, T.W. Light in tiny holes. *Nature* **2007**, *445*, 39–46.
8. Ding, Y.; Jiang, Z.; Saha, K.; Kim, C.S.; Kim, S.T.; Landis, R.F.; Rotello, V.M. Gold Nanoparticles for Nucleic Acid Delivery. *Mol. Ther.* **2014**, *22*, 1075–1083.

9. Rezić, I.; Zeiner, M.; Steffan, I. Determination of 28 selected elements in textiles by axially viewed inductively coupled plasma optical emission spectrometry, *Talanta* **2011**, *83*, 865–871.
10. Hinterwirth, H.; Wiedmer, S.K.; Moilanen, M.; Lehner, A.; Allmaier, G.; Waitz, T.; Lindner, W.; Lämmerhofer, M. Comparative method evaluation for size and size-distribution analysis of gold nanoparticles. *J. Sep. Sci.* **2013**, *36*, 2952–2961.
11. World Health Organization, Antimicrobial Resistance Global Report on Surveillance. Available online: https://www.who.int/drugresistance/documents/surveillancereport/en/ (accessed on October the 2nd 2022).
12. Van Hal, S.J.; Jensen, S.O.; Vaska, V.L.; Espedido, B.A.; Paterson, D.L.; Gosbell, I.B. Predictors of mortality in Staphylococcus aureus bacteremia. *Clin. Microbiol. Rev.* **2012**, *25*, 362–386.
13. Arduino, J.M. DRPH Photo Credit: Janice Haney Carr Center for Disease Control Prevention's Public Health Image Library PHIL, ID #11157. Available online: https://phil.cdc.gov/Details.aspx?pid=11156 (accessed on October the 2nd 2022).
14. Hanberger, H.; Walther, S.; Leone, M.; Barie, P.S.; Rello, J.; Lipman, J.; Marshall, J.C.; Anzueto, A.; Sakr, Y.; Pickkers, P.; et al. Increased mortality associated with meticillin-resistant Staphylococcus aureus (MRSA) infection in the Intensive Care Unit: Results from the EPIC II study. *Int. J. Antimicrob. Agents* **2011**, *38*, 331–335.
15. Hiramatsu, K.; Aritaka, N.; Hanaki, H.; Kawasaki, S.; Hosoda, Y.; Hori, S.; Fukuchi, Y.; Kobayashi, I. Dissemination in Japanese hospitals of strains of Staphylococcus aureus heterogeneously resistant to vancomycin. *Lancet* **1997**, *350*, 1670–1673.
16. McCaig, L.F.; McDonald, L.C.; Mandal, S.; Jernigan, D.B. Staphylococcus aureus–associated skin and soft tissue infections in ambulatory care. *Emerg. Infect. Dis.* **2006**, *12*, 1715.
17. Wieneke, A.A.; Roberts, D.; Gilbert, R.J. Staphylococcal food poisoning in the United Kingdom, 1969–*Epidemiology Infect.* **1993**, *110*, 519–531.
18. Sheehy, S.; Atkins, B.; Bejon, P.; Byren, I.; Wyllie, D.; Athanasou, N.; Berendt, A.; McNally, M. The microbiology of chronic osteomyelitis: Prevalence of resistance to common empirical anti-microbial regimens. *J. Infect.* **2010**, *60*, 338–343.
19. Khatib, R.; Johnson, L.B.; Sharma, M.; Fakih, M.G.; Ganga, R.; Riederer, K. Persistent Staphylococcus aureus bacteremia: Incidence and outcome trends over time. *Scand. J. Infect. Dis.* **2009**, *41*, 4–9.
20. Fowler, V.G.; Miro, J.M.; Hoen, B.; Cabell, C.H.; Abrutyn, E.; Rubinstein, E.; Corey, G.R.; Spelman, D.; Bradley, S.F.; Barsic, B.; et

al. Staphylococcus aureus endocarditis: A consequence of medical progress. *JAMA* **2005**, *293*, 3012–3021.
21. Tong, S.Y.C.; Davis, J.S.; Eichenberger, E.; Holland, T.L.; Fowler, V.G., Jr. Staphylococcus aureus Infections: Epidemiology, Pathophysiology, Clinical Manifestations, and Management. *Clin. Microbiol. Rev.* **2015**, *28*, 603–661.
22. Ammerlaan, H.; Seifert, H.; Harbarth, S.; Brun-Buisson, C.; Torres, A.; Antonelli, M.; Kluytmans, J.; Bonten, M.; Study on European Practices of Infections with Staphylococcus aureus (SEPIA) Study Group Adequacy of Antimicrobial Treatment and Outcome of*Staphylococcus aureus*Bacteremia in 9 Western European Countries. *Clin. Infect. Dis.* **2009**, *49*, 997–1005.
23. Gotland, N.; Uhre, M.L.; Mejer, N.; Skov, R.; Petersen, A.; Larsen, A.R.; Benfield, T.; Danish Staphylococcal Bacteremia Study Group. Long-term mortality and causes of death associated with Staphylococcus aureus bacteremia. A matched cohort study. *J. Infect.* **2016**, *73*, 346–357.
24. Díez-Pascual, A.M. Antibacterial Activity of Nanomaterials. *Nanomaterials* **2018**, *8*, 359–365.
25. Ramos, M.A.D.S.; Da Silva, P.B.; Spósito, L.; De Toledo, L.G.; Bonifácio, B.V.; Rodero, C.F.; Dos Santos, K.C.; Chorilli, M.; Bauab, T.M. Nanotechnology-based drug delivery systems for control of microbial biofilms: A review. *Int. J. Nanomed.* **2018**, *13*, 1179.
26. Al-Dhabi, N.A.; Mohammed Ghilan, A.K.; Arasu, M.V. Characterization of silver nanomaterials derived from marine Streptomyces sp. al-dhabi-87 and its in vitro application against multidrug resistant and extended-spectrum beta-lactamase clinical pathogens. *Nanomaterials* **2018**, *8*, 279.
27. Wijnhoven, S.W.; Peijnenburg, W.J.; Herberts, C.A.; Hagens, W.I.; Oomen, A.G.; Heugens, E.H.; Roszek, B.; Bisschops, J.; Gosens, I.; Van De Meent, D.; et al. Nano-silver—A review of available data and knowledge gaps in human and environmental risk assessment. *Nanotoxicology* **2009**, *3*, 109–138.
28. Blecher, K.; Nasir, A.; Friedman, A. The growing role of nanotechnology in combating infectious disease. *Virulence* **2011**, *2*, 395–401.
29. Huh, A.J.; Kwon, Y.J. "Nanoantibiotics": A new paradigm for treating infectious diseases using nanomaterials in the antibiotics resistant era. *J. Control. Release* **2011**, *156*, 128–145.

30. Shah, M.A.; Ahmad, T. *Principles of Nanoscience and Nanotechnology*; Alpha Science International: London, UK; Oxford, UK, 2010; pp. 10–20.
31. Pelgrift, R.Y.; Friedman, A.J. Nanotechnology as a therapeutic tool to combat microbial resistance. *Adv. Drug Deliv. Rev.* **2013**, *65*, 1803–1815.
32. Abramovitz, I.; Wisblech, D.; Zaltsman, N.; Weiss, E.I.; Beyth, N. Intratubular Antibacterial Effect of Polyethyleneimine Nanoparticles: An *Ex Vivo*Study in Human Teeth. *J. Nanomater.* **2015**, *2015*, 1–5.
33. Stoimenov, P.K.; Klinger, R.L.; Marchin, G.L.; Klabunde, K.J. Metal Oxide Nanoparticles as Bactericidal Agents. *Langmuir* **2002**, *18*, 6679–6686.
34. Magiorakos, A.P.; Srinivasan, A.; Carey, R.B.; Carmeli, Y.; Falagas, M.E.; Giske, C.G.; Harbarth, S.; Hindler, J.F.; Kahlmeter, G.; Olsson-Liljequist, B.; et al. Multidrug-resistant, extensively drug-resistant prug-resistant bacteria: An international expert proposal for interim stard definitions for acquired resistance. *Clin. Microbiol. Infect.* **2012**, *183*, 268–281.
35. Varner, K.E.; El-Badawy, A.; Feldhake, D.; Venkatapathy, R. *State-of-the-Science Review: Everything Nanosilver and More*; US Environmental Protection Agency: Washington, DC, USA, 2010.
36. Kesić, A.; Horozić, E. Prednosti i neželjeni efekti primjene metalnih nanočestica i metalnih oksida u farmaceutskim i kozmetičkim preparatima. *Šesti Međunarodni Kongr. Biomed. I Geonauke-Utic. Zivotn. Sred. Na Zdr. Ljud.* **2016**, 1, 218–225.
37. Sehmi, S.K.; Noimark, S.D.; Pike, S.; Bear, J.C.; Peveler, W.J.; Williams, C.K.; Shaffer, M.; Allan, E.; Parkin, I.P.; MacRobert, A.J. Enhancing the Antibacterial Activity of Light-Activated Surfaces Containing Crystal Violet and ZnO Nanoparticles: Investigation of Nanoparticle Size, Capping Ligand, and Dopants. *ACS Omega* **2016**, *1*, 334–343.
38. Panáček, A.; Kvítek, L.; Smékalová, M.; Večeřová, R.; Kolář, M.; Röderová, M.; Dyčka, F.; Šebela, M.; Prucek, R.; Tomanec, O.; et al. Bacterial resistance to silver nanoparticles and how to overcome it. *Nat. Nanotechnol.* **2017**, *13*, 65–71.
39. Grohmann, E. Available online: https://prof.beuth-hochschule.de/grohmann/ (accessed on September 30th 2022).
40. Shkodra-Pula, B.; Vollrath, A.; Schubert, U.S.; Schubert, S. Polymer-based nanoparticles for biomedical applications. In *Frontiers of Nanoscience*; Elsevier: Amsterdam, The Netherlands, 2020; Volume 16, pp. 233–252. ISBN: 978-0-08-102828-5.

41. Franco, D.; Calabrese, G.; Guglielmino, S.P.P.; Conoci, S. Metal-Based Nanoparticles: Antibacterial Mechanisms and Biomedical Application. *Microorganisms* **2022**, *10*, 1778. https://doi.org/10.3390/microorganisms10091778.
42. Unuma, H.; Hirose, Y.; Ito, M.; Watanabe, K. Preparation of the Precursor of Porous Alumina Particles using Immobilized Urease in Alginate Gel Templates. *J. Ceram. Soc. Jpn.* **2004**, *112*, 409–411.
43. Unuma, H.; Matsushima, Y.; Kawai, T. Enzyme-mediated synthesis of ceramic materials. *J. Ceram. Soc. Jpn.* **2011**, *119*, 623–630.
44. Li, X.; Xu, H.; Chen, Z.-S.; Chen, G. Biosynthesis of Nanoparticles by Microorganisms and Their Applications. *J. Nanomater.* **2011**, *2011*, 1–16.
45. Mandal, D.; Bolander, M.E.; Mukhopadhyay, D.; Sarkar, G.; Mukherjee, P. The use of microorganisms for the formation of metal nanoparticles and their application. *Appl. Microbiol. Biotechnol.* **2006**, *69*, 485–492.
46. Stoddart, A. Enzyme catalysis. *Nat. Mater.* **2012**, *11*, 910–910.
47. Chen, L.; Shen, Y.; Xie, A.; Huang, B.; Jia, R.; Guo, R.; Tang, W. Bacteria-Mediated Synthesis of Metal Carbonate Minerals with Unusual Morphologies and Structures. *Cryst. Growth Des.* **2008**, *9*, 743–754.
48. Sondi, I.; Matijević, E. Homogeneous Precipitation of Calcium Carbonates by Enzyme Catalyzed Reaction. *J. Colloid Interface Sci.* **2001**, *238*, 208–214.
49. Sondi, I.; Matijević, E. Homogeneous Precipitation by Enzyme Catalyzed Reactions. II. Strontium Barium Carbonates. *Chem. Mater.* **2003**, *15*, 1322–1326.
50. Zhao, J.; Sekikawa, H.; Kawai, T.; Unuma, H. Ferrimagnetic magnetite hollow microspheres prepared via enzymatically precipitated iron hydroxide on a urease-bearing polymer template. *J. Ceram. Soc. Jpn.* **2009**, *117*, 344–346.
51. Kawashita, M.; Takayama, Y.; Kokubo, T.; Takaoka, G.H.; Araki, N.; Hiraoka, M. Enzymatic Preparation of Hollow Yttrium Oxide Microspheres for In Situ Radiotherapy of Deep-Seated Cancer. *J. Am. Ceram. Soc.* **2006**, *89*, 1347–1351.
52. Hamaya, T.; Takizawa, T.; Hidaka, H.; Horikoshi, K. A new method for the preparation of magnetic alginate beads.. *J. Chem. Eng. Jpn.* **1993**, *26*, 223–224.
53. Kato, S.; Makino, T.; Unuma, H.; Takahashi, M. Enzyme Catalyzed Preparation of Hollow Alumina Precursor Using Emulsion Template.. *J. Ceram. Soc. Jpn.* **2001**, *109*, 369–371.

54. Kato, S.; Unuma, H.; Ota, T.; Takahashi, M. Homogeneous Precipitation of Hydrous Tin Oxide Powders at Room Temperature Using Enzymatically Induced Gluconic Acid as a Precipitant. *J. Am. Ceram. Soc.* **2004**, *83*, 986–988.
55. Yeom, B.; Char, K. Nanostructured $CaCO_3$ Thin Films Formed on the Urease Multilayers Prepared by the Layer-by-Layer Deposition. *Chem. Mater.* **2009**, *22*, 101–107.
56. Kawai, T.; Sekikawa, H.; Unuma, H. Preparation of hollow hydroxyapatite microspheres utilizing poly(divinylbenzene) as a template. *J. Ceram. Soc. Jpn.* **2009**, *117*, 340–343.
57. Kawashita, M.; Sadaoka, K.; Kokubo, T.; Saito, T.; Takano, M.; Araki, N.; Hiraoka, M. Enzymatic preparation of hollow magnetite microspheres for hyperthermic treatment of cancer. *J. Mater. Sci. Mater. Med.* **2006**, *17*, 605–610.
58. Malel, E.; Ludwig, R.; Gorton, L.; Madnler, D. Local Deposition of Au Nanpoarticles by Direct Electron Transfer through Cellobiose Dehydrogenase, *Chem. A Eur. J.* **2010**, *16*, 11697–1706.
59. Rodrigues-Lorenzo, L.; Rica, R.; Alvarez-Puebla, R.A.; Liz-Marzan, L.M. Plasmonic nanosensors with inverse sensitivity by means of enzyme guided crystal growth, *Nat. Mater.* **2012**, *11*, 604–607.
60. Allmaier, G.; Bacher, G.; Kaufman, S.L.; Szymanski, W.W. Molecular mass determination of noncovalent complexes biopolymers—proteins carbohydrates–by applying a gas-phase electrophoretic mobility mass analyzer. *J.* Aerosol *Sci.* **1999**, *30*, S303–S304.
61. Allmaier, G.; Laschober, C.; Reischl, G.P.; Szymanski, W.W. Austrian Patent Surgical Cutting and Fastening Instrument with Closure Trigger Locking Mechanism, 502 207 A1 2007 02 Patent, 15 February 2007.
62. Allmaier, G.; Laschober, C.; Szymanski, W.W. 2008 Nano ES GEMMA nad PDMA, New Tools for the Analysis of Nanobioparticles–Protein Complexes, Lipoparticles, Viruses. *J. Am. Soc. Mass Spectrom.* **2008**, *19*, 1062–1068.
63. Kallinger, P.; Weiss, V.; Lehner, A.; Allmaier, G.; Szymanski, W. Analysis hling of bio-nanoparticles environmental nanoparticles using electrostatic aerosol mobility. *Particuology* **2013**, *11*, 14–19.
64. Rezić, I.; Rezić, T.; Bokić, L. Optimization of the TLC separation of seven amino acids. *J. Planar Chromatogr. Mod. TLC* **2007**, *20*, 173–177.
65. Rezić, I. Rezić I.; Majdak M.; Kirin, P.; Vinceković, M.; Jurić, S.; Sopko S.; Vlahoviček Kahlina K.; Somogyi Škoc, M. Functionalized Microcapsules With Silver For Medical Textiles // 14th Scientific-

Professional Symposium Textile Science And Economy: Book of abstracts, Zagreb: Tekstilno-tehnološki fakultet, 2022. 3, 8
66. Rezić, I. Prediction of the surface tension of surfactant mixtures for detergent formulation using Design Expert software. **2011**, *142*, 1219–1225.
67. Rezić, I. Somogyi Škoc, M.; Pokrovac, I. Ljoljić Bilić, V.; Kosalec, I. Characterization of materials with nanoparticles and their biological and environmental impact // Proceedings of 141ST Iastem International Conference / International Academy Of Science, Technology, Engineering And Management, 2018. 54-57
68. Rezić, I.; Ćurković, L.; Ujević, M. Simple methods for characterization of metals in historical textile threads. *Talanta* **2010**, *82*, 237–244.
69. Rezić, I.; Ćurković, L.; Ujević, M. Study of microstructure and corrosion kinetic of steel guitar strings in artificial sweat solution. *Mater. Corros.* **2010**, *61*, 524–529.
70. Rezić, I.; Steffan, I. ICP-OES determination of metals present in textile materials. *Microchem. J.* **2007**, *85*, 46–51.
71. Rezić, I. Optimization of ultrasonic extraction of 23 elements from cotton. *Ultrason. Sonochem.* **2009**, *16*, 63–69.
72. Rezić, I.; Rolich, T. Artificial neural networks in chromatography spectroscopy. In *Artificial Neural Networks*; Nova Science Publishers: New York, NY, USA, 2011, pp. 123–138.
73. Rezić, I. Thin layer chromatographic monitoring of sonolytic degradation of surfactants in wastewaters. *J. Planar Chromatogr. Mod. TLC* **2019**, *26*, 96–101.
74. Reich, E.S. Ultimate upgrade for US synchrotron. *Nature* **2013**, *501*, 148–149.
75. Schmitt, B.; Brönnimann, C.; Eikenberry, E.F.; Gozzo, F.; Hörmann, C.; Horisberger, R.; Patterson, B. Mythen detector system. *Nucl. Instrum. Methods Phys. Res. A* **2003**, *501*, 267–239.
76. Brönnimann, C.; Baur, R.; Eikenberry, E.F.; Kohout, S.; Lindner, M.; Schmitt, B.; Horisberger, R. A pixel read-out chip for the PILATUS project. *Nucl. Instrum. Methods Phys. Res. A* **2001**, *465*, 235–272.
77. Petkov, V.; Peng, Y.; Williams, G.; Huang, B.; Tomalia, D.; Ren, Y. Structure of gold nanoparticles suspended in water studied by x-ray diffraction and computer simulations. *Phys. Rev. B* **2005**, *72*, 195402.
78. Jacques, S.D.M.; Di Michiel, M.; Kimber, S.A.J.; Yang, X.; Cernik, R.J.; Beale, A.M.; Billinge, S.J.L. Pair distribution function computed tomography. *Nat. Commun.* **2013**, *4*, 2536.

79. Sherma, B.; Mani, S.; Sarma, T.K. Biogenic Growth of Alloys Core Shell Nanostructures Using Urease as a Nanoreactor at Ambient Conditions. *Nat. Sci. Rep.* **2013**, *3*, 1–8.
80. De la Rica, R.; Matsui, H.; Urease as a Nanoreactor for Growing Crystalline ZnO Nanoshells at Room Temperature. *Angewte Chem. Int. Ed.* **2008**, *47*, 5415–5417.
81. Granquist, C.G. Transparent conductors as solar energy materials: A panoramic review. *Sol. Energy Mater. Sol. Cells* **2007**, *91*, 1529–1598.
82. Ebbesen, T.W.; Lezec, H.J.; Ghaemi, H.F.; Thio, T.; Wolff, P.A. Extraordinary optical transmission through sub-wavelength hole arrays. *Nature* **1998**, *391*, 667–669.
83. Martinaga Pintarić, L.; Somogi Škoc, M.; Ljoljić Bilić, V.; Pokrovac, I.; Kosalec, I.; Rezić, I. Synthesis, modification and characterization of antimicrobial textile surface containing ZnO nanoparticles. *Polymers* **2020**, *12*, 1210.
84. Rezić, I.; Majdak, M.; Bilić, V.L.; Pokrovac, I.; Martinaga, L.; Škoc, M.S.; Kosalec, I. Development of Antibacterial Protective Coatings Active against MSSA and MRSA on Biodegradable Polymers. *Polymers* **2021**, *13*, 659.
85. Rezić, I.; Somogyi Škoc, M.; Majdak, M.; Jurić, S.; Stracenski, K.S.; Vinceković, M. Functionalization of Polymer Surface with Antimicrobial Microcapsules. *Polymers* **2022**, *14*, 1961.
86. Rezić, I.; Škoc, M.S.; Majdak, M.; Jurić, S.; Stracenski, K.S.; Vlahoviček-Kahlina, K.; Vinceković, M. ICP-MS Determination of Antimicrobial Metals in Microcapsules. *Molecules* **2022**, *27*, 3219.
87. Vukoja, D.; Vlainić, J.; Ljolić Bilić, V.; Martinaga, L.; Rezić, I.; Brlek Gorski, D.; Kosalec, I. Innovative Insights into In Vitro Activity of Colloidal Platinum Nanoparticles against ESBL-Producing Strains of Escherichia coli and Klebsiella pneumoniae. *Pharmaceutics* **2022**, *14*, 1714.
88. Rezić, I.; Kracher, D.; Oros, D.; Mujadžić, S.; Anđelini, M.; Kurtanjek, Ž.; Ludwig, R.; Rezić, T. Application of Causality Modelling for Prediction of Molecular Properties for Textile Dyes Degradation by LPMO. *Molecules* **2022**, *27*, 6390.
89. Egbuna, C.; Parmar, V.K.; Jeevanandam, J.; Ezzat, S.M.; Patrick-Iwuanyanwu, K.C.; Adetunji, C.O.; Khan, J.; Onyeike, E.N.; Uche, C.Z.; Akram, M.; et al. Toxicity of Nanoparticles in Biomedical Application: Nanotoxicology. *J. Toxicol.* **2021**, *2021*, 1–21.
90. Blanco-Andujar, C.; Thanh, N.T. Synthesis of nanoparticles for biomedical applications. *Annu. Rep. Sect. A Inorg. Chem.* **2010**, *106*, 553–568.

91. Uthaman, A.; Lal, H.; Thomas, S. Fundamentals of Silver Nanoparticles and Their Toxicological Aspects. In *Polymer Nanocomposites Based on Silver Nanoparticles. Engineering Materials*; Lal, H.M., Thomas, S., Li, T., Maria, H.J., Eds.; Springer: Cham, Switzerland, 2021; pp. 1–24.
92. Dikshit, P.K.; Kumar, J.; Das, A.K.; Sadhu, S.; Sharma, S.; Singh, S.; Gupta, P.K.; Kim, B.S. Green synthesis of metallic nanoparticles: Applications and limitations. *Catalysts* **2021**, *11*, 902.
93. De Silva, C.; Nawawi, N.M.; Abd Karim, M.M.; Abd Gani, S.; Masarudin, M.J.; Gunasekaran, B.; Ahmad, S.A. The mechanistic action of biosynthesised silver nanoparticles and its application in aquaculture and livestock industries. *Animals* **2021**, *11*, 2097.
94. Xu, L.; Yi-Yi, W.; Huang, J.; Chun-Yuan, C.; Zhen-Xing, W.; Xie, H. Silver nanoparticles: Synthesis, medical applications and biosafety. *Theranostics* **2020**, *10*, 8996–9031.
95. Almatroudi, A. Silver nanoparticles: Synthesis, characterisation and biomedical applications. *Open Life Sci.* **2020**, *15*, 819–839.
96. Barani, H.; Mahltig, B. Microwave-assisted synthesis of silver nanoparticles: Effect of reaction temperature and precursor concentration on fluorescent property. *J. Clust. Sci.* **2020**, 1, 1–11. https://doi.org/10.1007/s10876-020-01945.
97. Patil, A.H.; Jadhav, S.A.; More, V.B.; Sonawane, K.D.; Patil, P.S. Novel one step sonosynthesis and deposition technique to prepare silver nanoparticles coated cotton textile with antibacterial properties. *Colloid J.* **2019**, *81*, 720–727.
98. Kuntyi, O.; Shepida, M.; Sozanskyi, M.; Sukhatskiy, Y.; Mazur, A.; Kytsya, A.; Bazylyak, L. Sonoelectrochemical synthesis of silver nanoparticles in sodium polyacrylate solution. *Biointerface Res. Appl. Chem.* **2021**, *11*, 12202–12214.
99. Seku, K.; Gangapuram, B.R.; Pejjai, B.; Kadimpati, K.K.; Golla, N. Microwave-assisted synthesis of silver nanoparticles and their application in catalytic, antibacterial and antioxidant activities. *J. Nanostructure Chem.* **2018**, *8*, 179–188.
100. Tola, O.H.; Oluwole, O.I.; Omotayo, A.B. Synthesis and characterization of silver nanoparticles from ecofriendly materials: A review. *Int. J. Eng. Res. Technol.* **2020**, *9*, 782–795.
101. Naganthran, A.; Verasoundarapandian, G.; Khalid, F.E.; Masarudin, M.J.; Zulkharnain, A.; Nawawi, N.M.; Karim, M.; Abdullah, C.A.C.; Ahmad, S.A. Synthesis, Characterization and Biomedical Application of Silver Nanoparticles. *Materials* **2022**, *15*, 427.

CHAPTER TWO

GREEN MEDICAL ANTIMICROBIAL NANOTOOLS[1]

Introduction

In this chapter, we delve into the realm of textile surface modification through the innovative sol–gel methodology. The focus here lies on an intriguing antimicrobial coating, infused with nanoparticles that exhibit potent antibacterial properties against antibiotic-resistant bacteria. As we traverse this chapter, we'll explore the interplay of various factors: ultrasonic irradiation power (ranging from 40 to 90 kHz), reagent concentrations (nanoparticles, precursor, and acids), and time spans (spanning from 15 to 72 minutes). These variables are intricately linked to the structural, morphological, and antimicrobial characteristics of coatings adorned with zinc oxide nanoparticles.

> Sol gel procedure is one of the most common techniques due to its numerous advantages. Among all it enables achieving flat and flexible surfaces, homogenous antimicrobial layer and a possibility of producing huge number of materials with novel coatings. Together with the antimicrobial effects, other advisable properties such are hydrophobicity, antiviral structure and UV protection are easily achieved.

The connection between sonocatalytic performance and the resulting modification's structure was established through a comprehensive array of techniques. These methods included FTIR spectroscopy (FTIR), scanning electron microscopy with an EDX detector (SEM-EDX), thin-layer chromatography (TLC), and an assessment of antimicrobial effects on specific model microorganisms. Notably, the uniformity of layers containing ZnO nanoparticles on the samples was markedly enhanced by

---

[1] L. Martinaga Pintarić, M. Somogi Škoc, V. Ljoljić Bilić, I. Pokrovac, I. Kosalec, I. Rezić*, Synthesis, Modification and Characterization of Antimicrobial Textile Surface Containing ZnO Nanoparticles, Polymers, 12 (2020) 1210; doi:10.3390/polym12061210, 1-15

amplifying both ultrasonic irradiation power and duration. This ultrasonic treatment yielded dual benefits: it not only harmonized the structure and morphology of the samples but also acted as a deterrent to nanoparticle agglomeration. In addition, the optimal conditions yielded a remarkable outcome: an antimicrobial coating infused with ZnO nanoparticles, exhibiting robust activity against bacterial strains like S. aureus and E. coli, was effectively synthesized.

Antimicrobial resistance

According to certain projections, the year 2050 could witness a startling reality: infections stemming from antibiotic-resistant bacteria might eclipse cancer as a leading cause of mortality. In Europe alone, the statistics paint a grim picture—approximately 25,000 lives are lost each year, with a financial burden exceeding EUR 1.5 billion, all attributed to the menace of resistant microorganisms [1]. Within this harrowing context, certain bacterial strains loom large as formidable adversaries. One such example is methicillin-resistant Staphylococcus aureus (MRSA), often referred to as a *"super-bacteria."* Its mounting defiance stems from an increasing resistance to an extensive spectrum of antibiotic-based penicillin medications, specifically the β-lactam antibiotics. Staphylococcus aureus belongs to the Gram-positive bacteria of spherical morphology, falling under the Staphylococcaceae family. Its impact on global health is profound, being among the most consequential pathogens.

The frequency of *Staphylococcus aureus* infections ranges from 20 to 50 cases per 100,000 individuals annually. Alarmingly, a grim fatality rate accompanies these infections, with mortality ranging from 10% to 30%. Remarkably, this toll surpasses the cumulative deaths attributed to a trio of formidable adversaries: *Acquired Immunodeficiency Syndrome* (AIDS), tuberculosis, and viral hepatitis. [1, 2].

Metal oxide nanoparticles exhibit remarkable attributes such as potent antimicrobial efficacy, water resistance, and robust protective qualities. In this realm, ZnO nanoparticles emerge as a pivotal player, standing out as a vital antimicrobial agent. This distinction underscores the integration of ZnO nanoparticle-coated cellulose materials within a diverse array of protective products. The exceptional antimicrobial prowess displayed by ZnO nanoparticles has garnered considerable worldwide attention. This heightened interest stems from the nanoparticles' diminutive diameters, which fall well below the dimensions of microorganisms. This unique characteristic is pivotal in conferring the pronounced antimicrobial activity that ZnO nanoparticles exhibit, further emphasizing their significance in this domain.

Recent research endeavors have unveiled intriguing insights into the interactions involving nanosized ZnO, shedding light on its antimicrobial mechanism. Notably, these nanoparticles can engage with bacterial surfaces and penetrate bacterial cells by traversing their membranes [3]. The versatility of ZnO nanoparticles' antimicrobial effects is noteworthy, extending their impact across a spectrum of microorganisms. This encompassing range includes both Gram-positive and Gram-negative bacteria, as well as hardy spores resilient to elevated temperatures and pressures [4]. Interestingly, despite their potent antimicrobial properties, ZnO nanoparticles exhibit a reassuring trait—they are non-toxic to human cells. This remarkable biocompatibility with human cells has been substantiated through the meticulous investigation conducted by Padmavathy and Vijayaraghavan [5]. Furthermore, ZnO's safety profile and compatibility with human skin render it a suitable candidate for incorporation into textiles and surfaces that come into contact with the human body [6,7]. This dual attribute positions ZnO nanoparticles as compelling antimicrobial agents with significant potential, warranting thorough exploration. Ongoing research endeavors are currently unraveling the full scope of their capabilities. It's worth noting that ZnO nanoparticles have demonstrated their antimicrobial efficacy across a broad spectrum of bacterial species, as corroborated by numerous researchers. [2,4,5,8–16].

Padmavathy and Vijayaraghavan investigated the antibacterial activity of ZnO nanoparticles with various particle sizes and reported that with a decreasing particle size the antibacterial efficiency of ZnO nanoparticles increased [5]. In this research, Gram-negative bacteria seemed to be more resistant to ZnO nanoparticles than Gram-positive bacteria, and the antibacterial activity of ZnO nanoparticles increased with decreasing particle size and increasing powder concentration. Moreover, the antibacterial effect of ZnO nanoparticles was time dependent.

ZnO nanoparticles hold unique optical, chemical sensing, semiconducting, electric conductivity, and piezoelectric properties [17], as well as high catalytic and high photochemical activities. ZnO's high optical absorption in the UVA and UVB regions (315–400/280–315 nm), is used as a UV protection [18]. Currently, the market for protective and medical antibacterial textiles is constrained by the elevated costs associated with such materials. This limitation has spurred a quest for innovative technologies that can revolutionize the production of antibacterial materials. While various pioneering methods have been explored, they have yet to achieve widespread adoption due to their intricate processes and resulting high price points.

In this landscape, ultrasonic irradiation emerges as a crucial component in the quest to embed antibacterial particles within modified textile materials. The application of ultrasonic irradiation plays a pivotal role in facilitating the incorporation of antimicrobial nanoparticles into polymer materials. Notably, Abramova and colleagues embarked on a notable endeavor wherein they employed the sol–gel methodology to synthesize titanium dioxide nanoparticles alongside zinc oxide nanoparticles. This synergistic approach utilized titanyl sulfate and zinc nitrate hexahydrate as precursors, aiming to evaluate the feasibility of generating antibacterial coatings on textile materials. While challenges persist in the pursuit of cost-effective antibacterial solutions, the integration of ultrasonic irradiation and nanoparticle modification underscores a promising avenue in the evolution of advanced textiles with enhanced protective properties. [19].

Reduction in the number of microorganisms of *Escherichia coli* by was more than 99.99% [19] Akhavan and Montazer loaded TiO_2 on cotton [20, 21]. They achieved excellent self-cleaning and UV-protection. In addition, the mechanical properties of nanocomposite films can be improved by ultrasonic irradiation [22]. Moreover, the addition of reducing, stabilizing and binding agents such as the natural biopolymer Tragacanth gum can benefit the *in situ* synthesis of zinc oxide nanoparticles on the cotton fabric. Ultrasonic synthesis of zinc oxide nanoparticles was done in a short time and at a low temperature [23]. The finished cotton fabric has efficient antimicrobial protection against *Staphylococcus aureus, Escherichia coli* and *Candida albicans*, with inhibition zones of 3.3 ± 0.1, 3.1 ± 0.1 and 3.0 ± 0.1 mm [23]. The modification of the morphology of ZnO nanoparticles, for example, into thorn-like ZnO nanoparticles, shows even more promising antimicrobial results [24]. The toxicity effects of nanomaterials are intricately influenced by factors such as particle composition, size, and shape. Understanding the intricate interplay of these elements is pivotal in comprehending the potential harm posed by nanoparticles. One of the central mechanisms underlying nanoparticle toxicity hinges on the generation of oxidative species. These reactive entities can inflict damage upon vital cellular components, including proteins and DNA. Furthermore, the catalytic, optical, and electrical properties of cells can also be adversely impacted by these oxidative species.

In the realm of nanoparticle toxicity investigation, specific biological defense mechanisms come into play to counter the effects of oxidative stress. Catalase, glutathione, and superoxide dismutase, as highlighted by Barata and colleagues, emerge as critical players in this defense system. These elements work in tandem to counteract the damaging impact of oxidative stress, underscoring the intricate cellular responses that contribute to our understanding of nanoparticle toxicity. [25]. Liu et al. proved that nanoparticles of ZnO, CuO, TiO_2, and Au are toxic to the daphnids of Daphnia magna and early life stages of zebrafish [26]. Mostly nanoparticles with diameters of 30 nm (ZnO) and 20 nm (TiO_2) induced more toxicity than larger dimensions (50 nm ZnO and 30 nm TiO_2) because smaller particles were more likely to enter the cell. The toxicological effects of ZnO nanoparticles are very important for cellulose materials, which are coming into direct contact with human skin. Therefore, this emphasizes the need for the intense investigation of ZnO nanoparticles and their effects on living organisms, including microorganisms [27].

Cellulose materials can be functionalized by applying layers of different nanoparticles to their structure. The functionalization of textiles with ZnO nanostructures enables the production of reinforced textiles resistant to tear and make wearing antibacterial textiles, UV- blocking textiles and other interesting materials possible. In addition to antibacterial properties, anti-odor, self-cleaning and medicinal textiles are made with ZnO. Functionalization can be achieved through different modifications, and the sol–gel process is an important part of them by being a simple, practical and cost-effective approach [28]. Moreover, it enables facile coating by obtaining a homogenous layer on large sample surfaces, the easy control of reaction kinetics, lower sintering temperatures and other advantages [28–30]. The most important advantages of the sol–gel process is the fact that a homogenous, unified and flat coating can be achieved at a mild and low temperature (below 100 °C), its flexibility and large surface modification [31].

Antimicrobial modification

This chapter will present modification of viscose and cellulose polymers (ISO 1833: 2003), with a mass per unit area of 72.26 g/m2 (EN ISO 2286-2:2008), 0.51 mm thickness (EN ISO 5084: 2003) and with 54 (50) threads/cm in warp (weft), respectively (EN 1049-2: 2003). All used chemicals were of analytical grade and were utilized without additional purification.

> Samples for modification can be made of any woven or non-woven textiles, polymer flat surfaces or 3D printed biopolymers

In the pursuit of enhancing cellulose materials, a dip-coating methodology was employed to introduce ZnO nanoparticles. The process leveraged 3-glycidyloxypropyltrimethoxysilane (GLYMO) from Sigma Aldrich, based in Darmstadt, Germany, Europe, serving as a precursor. The coating process was executed at a controlled speed of 1 mm/s. The procedure commenced by subjecting ZnO nanoparticle-laden sols to magnetic stirring. Subsequently, GLYMO was introduced, initiating a series of steps involving ultrasonic irradiation at various intensity levels and time intervals. This intricate sequence persisted until a state of uniformity within the solution was achieved. After allowing the samples to undergo gelation at room temperature, a subsequent drying phase was orchestrated. The samples were subjected to a 24-hour drying period at room temperature under atmospheric pressure, followed by a subsequent exposure to 100 °C for 60 minutes. To assess the efficacy of the cellulose modification process, a battery of analytical techniques was brought into play. Thin layer chromatography (TLC) facilitated the characterization of the modified products, offering insights into their composition. Meanwhile, scanning electron microscopy with an EDX detector (SEM-EDX), facilitated by Tescan Vega of Brno, Czech Republic, unveiled the morphological details and elemental composition of the modified cellulose. Additionally, FTIR-ATR spectroscopy, conducted using equipment from Perkin Elmer in Waltham, Massachusetts, USA, enabled a deeper understanding of the molecular structure and interactions present within the modified materials. Throughout this intricate endeavor, the sol–gel process was subjected to meticulous optimization. A myriad of influential parameters—ranging from temperature and time to the role of the precursor and HCl as a catalyst—were systematically fine-tuned to achieve an optimal outcome in this multifaceted process. (Figure 2.1.).

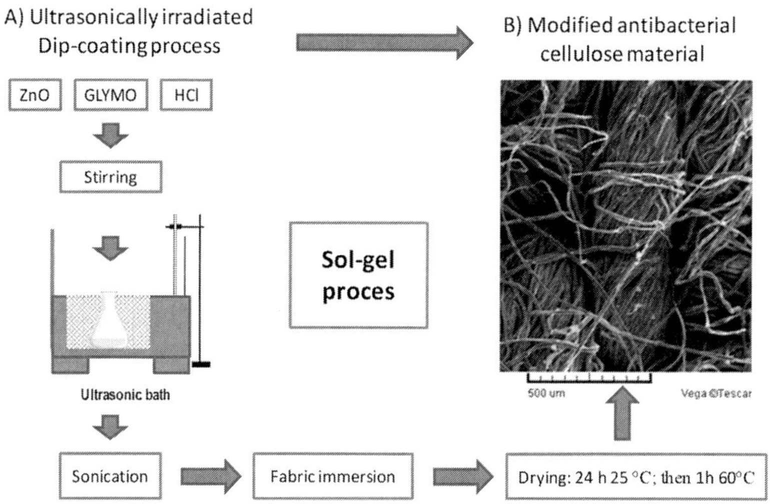

Figure 2.1. Schematic overview of ultrasonically irradiated dip-coating process with

This chapter embarks on an extensive exploration, delving into the intricate influence of various parameters on the modification of cellulose materials with zinc oxide (ZnO) nanoparticles via the sol–gel method. Specifically, the interplay of ultrasonic irradiation power, reagent concentrations encompassing nanoparticles, organic precursor, and acid, alongside distinct time intervals, will be meticulously examined. The focus lies on understanding how these factors collectively shape the structure, morphology, and antimicrobial attributes of the modified cellulose.

To unveil the transformative effects of this modification process, comprehensive characterization techniques were employed. The scanning electron microscope "TESCAN VEGA TS5136LS," hailing from Tescan Vega company in Brno, Czech Republic, emerged as a pivotal tool. Augmented with an Energy Dispersive X-ray Spectroscopy (EDS) detector, this instrument facilitated the observation of sample structure and morphology both before and after ZnO nanoparticle modification.

Further insight into the material's transformation was gleaned through Fourier transform infrared spectroscopy (FTIR). Employing the Spectrum 100 FTIR apparatus from Perkin Elmer, stationed in Waltham, Massachusetts, U.S.A., this analysis harnessed KBr and Attenuated Total Reflectance (ATR) techniques. This enabled the probing of functional groups present in cellulose materials pre and post modification. Spectra were meticulously recorded in diffuse reflectance mode, spanning a frequency range from 400 to 4000 cm−1 at a resolution of 4cm−1. Notably, this methodology facilitated the identification of various functional groups and chemical structures within ZnO nanoparticles through the scrutiny of electromagnetic wave absorption at distinct frequencies and intensities. Peak identification entailed averaging three scans for each sample.

To comprehensively capture the dimensions and distribution of nanoparticles, a Nanoparticle Tracking Analyzer (NTA) named "Nanosight" was harnessed. This cutting-edge technology provided crucial insights into nanoparticle size and spatial distribution, further augmenting the overall understanding of the cellulose modification process.

Antimicrobial activity

In standardized testing systems, the samples of interest are investigated by disc-diffusion and growth inhibition studies against Gram-positive (*Staphylococcus aureus*) and Gram-negative (*Escherichia coli)* bacteria, and Funghi (*Candida albicans*). In order to assess the effects of ultrasonic irradiation on the antimicrobial effects of modified polymers, the *in vitro* antimicrobial activity of used colloidal ZnO nanoparticles for different model microorganisms were investigated by agar well diffusion and serial two-fold microdilution assays.

Optimization

In this chapter, the response surface methodology (RSM) based on Design of Experiment (State Ease version 9.1, State Ease Company, USA) software is described [35, 36]. D-optimal design was selected for obtaining optimal results with a minimal number of preliminary experiments [37,38]. After the selection of the design, a “candidate set” with selected points was generated.

Table 2.1. Investigated parameters used during optimization of dip-coating process by Design of Experiment statistical methodology and calculated recovery angles. Input parameters were concentration of GLYMO [1], 2 volume[2] of 0.1 M HCl, mass concentration of ZnO[3] per 100 mL, frequency of the ultrasound[4] and time in minutes[5].

Output was recovery angle, as a measure of flexibility after the treatment.

Nr	1	2	3	4	5	Output
1	45.0	41.8	0.70	67.5	45.0	132.6
2	45.0	78.2	0.70	67.5	45.0	126.6
3	45.0	60.0	0.70	67.5	45.0	117.7
4	50.0	70.0	0.40	55.0	60.0	121.7
5	35.9	60.0	0.70	67.5	45.0	112.8
6	40.0	70.0	1.00	55.0	60.0	130.7
7	45.0	60.0	0.70	67.5	17.7	128.8
8	40.0	70.0	0.40	80.0	60.0	129.3
9	45.0	60.0	0.70	44.7	45.0	136.2
10	45.0	60.0	0.15	67.5	45.0	129.2
11	45.0	60.0	0.70	90.3	45.0	133.2
12	45.0	60.0	0.70	67.5	45.0	128.2
13	50.0	70.0	1.00	55.0	30.0	125.5
14	45.0	60.0	0.70	67.5	45.0	133.5
15	40.0	50.0	0.40	55.0	30.0	130.1
16	50.0	50.0	1.00	55.0	60.0	130.6
17	45.0	60.0	0.70	67.5	45.0	131.6
18	45.0	60.0	0.70	67.5	72.3	126.1
19	45.0	60.0	0.70	67.5	45.0	131.3
20	50.0	50.0	0.40	80.0	60.0	137.5
21	40.0	70.0	1.00	80.0	30.0	138.8
22	54.1	60.0	0.70	67.5	45.0	134.6
23	45.0	60.0	1.25	67.5	45.0	138.2
24	40.0	50.0	1.00	80.0	60.0	138.8
25	50.0	50.0	1.00	80.0	30.0	137.5
26	50.0	70.0	0.40	80.0	30.0	133.0

The meticulous design of the experimental setup was underpinned by a systematic selection procedure. This process was informed by preliminary experiments that harnessed computer-intensive matrix modeling. The overarching goal was to attain an elevated level of precision within the model. In pursuit of this, a total of 26 preliminary experiments were meticulously devised and executed, as outlined in Table 2.1. The foundation for this modeling endeavor was established through the identification of initial parameters. These parameters encompassed time, temperature, ultrasonic irradiation power, and concentrations of essential reagents, namely, GLYMO, HCl, and ZnO nanoparticles. The strategic orchestration of these factors aimed to pave the way for a robust and intricately refined experimental framework. The ultimate objective was to uncover insights that could guide the optimal modification process for enhanced cellulose materials with ZnO nanoparticles.

> Only by applying sophisticated statistical methodology such is Design of Experiment; it is possible to investigate the interactions among process parameters. By this, hidden relationship among some variables can be detected even if variables per se do not have any influence on the system in progress.

The elastic behaviour of modified polymers was tested according to the norm, HRN EN ISO 22313: 2008, in which the material is exposed to the bending load at a 180° angle curve with the load on the press, released, and then the time needed to achieve the sample's original position is measured. For preliminary testing, in order to see which metals are present in the sample, thin-layer chromatography was applied. The standard sample solution was spotted on 20 × 20 cm TLC cellulose pre-coated plates (Merck, Darmstadt, Germany) by glass capillary. Development was, after the saturation of the chromatographic chamber, carried out in the Camag chromatographic chamber by the ascending technique to 8 cm distance. For the mobile system, acetonitrile–hydrochloric acid–water (72: 25: 23) was chosen. After development, the plates were dried, and exposed to ammonia vapours. The chromatograms with coloured spots occurred after 37 min of the development, and showed the presence of zinc. R_F factors for each metal was calculated by using the following calculation:

$$R_F = l_i/l_0$$

presenting the ration between the distances reached by the sample and the mobile phase. After testing the standard metal solutions, the solutions of samples were investigated in the same way.

The comprehensive modification process encompassed a multitude of influential parameters, each contributing to the desired properties. To enhance the efficiency of the sol–gel modification, the integration of concentrated HCl was employed. This strategic addition facilitated a more robust and effective transformation. Furthermore, achieving a uniform distribution of nanoparticles within the coating was made possible through ultrasonic homogenization—a technique that contributed to the consistent dispersion of nanoparticles. Central to this process was the utilization of the precursor 3-glycidyloxypropyltrimethoxysilane (GLYMO). This precursor underwent thorough characterization via FTIR spectroscopy and scanning electron microscopy equipped with an Energy Dispersive X-ray (EDX) detector (SEM-EDX). These analytical methods provided insights into the molecular and structural features of the GLYMO coating.

The focal point of this endeavor was the incorporation of ZnO nanoparticles. These nanoparticles, boasting certified particle sizes of less than 100nm, were meticulously chemically bonded to the cellulose surface. This intricate integration led to the creation of a functionalized cellulose material imbued with antibacterial attributes. The investigative phase involved a systematic exploration of the influence of ultrasonic irradiation power (ranging from 40 to 90 kHz), the concentrations of essential reagents (including nanoparticles, precursor, and acids), and the duration of the process (spanning from 15 to 72 minutes). This comprehensive analysis aimed to unravel the impact of these parameters on the resulting structure, morphology, and antimicrobial effectiveness of coatings enriched with zinc oxide nanoparticles. To assess the efficacy of this modified material, the antimicrobial effects of colloidal ZnO nanoparticles were evaluated against two reference bacterial strains, namely *Staphylococcus aureus (S. aureus*) and *Escherichia coli (E. coli*).

Additionally, the "killing effect" of cellulose materials modified with 100nm ZnO nanoparticles was gauged against both a methicillin-sensitive and a methicillin-resistant strain of *Staphylococcus aureus*. This comprehensive evaluation offered insights into the potential application and potency of the modified cellulose materials in combating bacterial pathogens. In this chapter, both SEM-EDX and FTIR spectroscopic methods were used to proof the quality of achieved modification of cellulose materials before the antimicrobial testing. SEM-EDX methodology enabled the fast and simple non-destructive investigation of the sample morphology and surface chemical composition [39–41]. The samples were observed under 80× magnification, after a process in which the samples were coated with the Au/Pd uniform coating (Figure 2.1).

The size of the colloidally stable ZnO nanoparticles used in the modification of cellulose materials for antimicrobial testing was investigated and monitored by the *Nanoparticle Tracking Analyzer Nanosight,* which can determine the concentration of nanoparticles, as well as their distribution in the system. All nanoparticles were 100–120 nm in size. Zinc monitored by thin-layer chromatography was determined under the R_F value of 0.16, and could be visualized by the pink color when detected with *Alizarin S* reagent. Secondly, the samples were investigated by Fourier-transform infrared spectrometry (Spectrum 100 FTIR, Perkin Elmer, Waltham, Massachusetts), which applies KBr and Attenuated Total Reflectance (ATR) techniques and enables the recording of the spectra of cellulose materials in their solid state (Figure 2). FTIR was applied as an excellent technique for the investigation of different solid samples [40], including cellulose samples before and after the modification with nanoparticles.

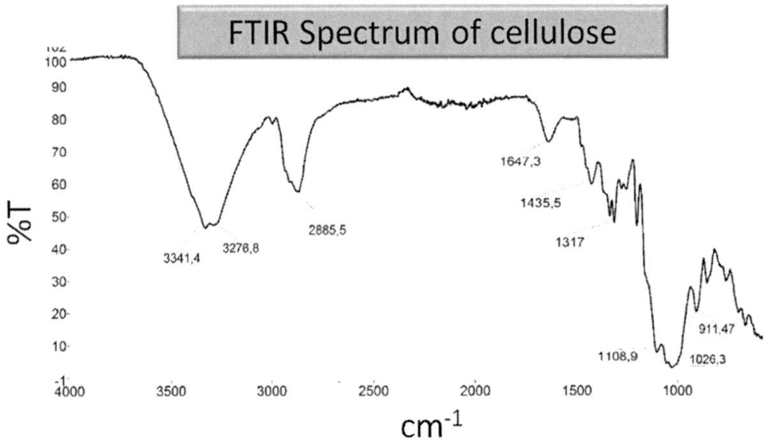

Figure 2.2. Fourier-transform infrared spectra of cellulose sample

Figure 2.2 reveals distinct disparities between the spectra of samples prior to and following the sol–gel modification process. These differences manifest in specific regions, each offering valuable insights into the underlying chemical transformations. The spectral features include noteworthy observations:

- **Epoxy Groups:** Evident around ~905 and 911 cm−1, these epoxy groups are indicative of specific molecular bonds. They play a key role in the reactivity of the precursor GLYMO. Notably, epoxy groups are known to selectively engage with primary amines and silanol moieties, thereby facilitating the intricate modification process.
- **Si–O Groups:** The area around 1100 cm−1 is intricately associated with Si–O groups, particularly Si–O–C and Si–O–Si bridges. This region signifies the presence of crucial bonds formed during the hydrolysis and crosslinking processes. These bonds contribute

significantly to the creation of a stable and functionalized cellulose material.

- **Conversion of Methyl Groups**: The transformation of methoxy groups within the precursor GLYMO is distinctly evident at ~2870 cm−1. This spectral feature underscores the dynamic alterations occurring during the modification process, shedding light on the molecular changes that contribute to the final product's properties.

Through a meticulous monitoring and optimization process, the hydrolysis and crosslinking reactions were navigated with precision. The overarching aim was to pinpoint the most favourable conditions that would culminate in the creation of an optimally efficient antimicrobial coating. These findings represent a pivotal step towards unlocking the potential of cellulose materials endowed with antimicrobial properties, broadening the horizons for their practical applications.

The quest for enhanced application properties prompted a deliberate focus on controlling the morphology of the inorganic phase within the hybrid structure. Achieving this was made possible through strategic adjustments to the hydrolysis conditions of GLYMO and other pertinent parameters. A well-recognized phenomenon emerged: hybrids originating from hydrolyzed GLYMO exhibited superior mechanical properties during acid hydrolysis. This unique attribute led to the formation of an exceptionally uniform hybrid structure—a crucial factor in enhancing the practical usability of the material. In the context of this research, hydrochloric acid (HCl) was harnessed as a catalyst to facilitate hydrolysis, thereby further refining the hybrid structure. However, it's important to note that the presence of hydrochloric acid does come at the cost of reduced thermal stability for these hybrids.

The reactivity of GLYMO in hydrolysis and condensation reactions is pivotal. During these processes, alkoxide groups and epoxy rings within GLYMO undergo opening reactions, culminating in the creation of covalent bonds. This intrinsic property underscores the material's potential as a foundational element in constructing hybrid materials characterized by strong organic-inorganic linkages.

Furthermore, the SEM-EDX results provided concrete evidence of the successful modification of cellulose materials. The SEM microphotograph in Figure 3a illustrates the surface with nanoparticle modification, and Figure 3b showcases the corresponding EDX spectra.

An intricate mapping of ZnO nanoparticles within a selected region is depicted in Figure 2.3. These visual representations validate the achievement of a uniform, homogenous coating (Figure 2.3.A) across the sample surface. Notably, the distribution of ZnO nanoparticles (Figure 2.3. B) is consistent and even, as evidenced by the mapping results in Figure 2.3c. This level of structural control signifies a significant accomplishment in tailoring cellulose materials for practical applications, particularly in the realm of antimicrobial coatings.

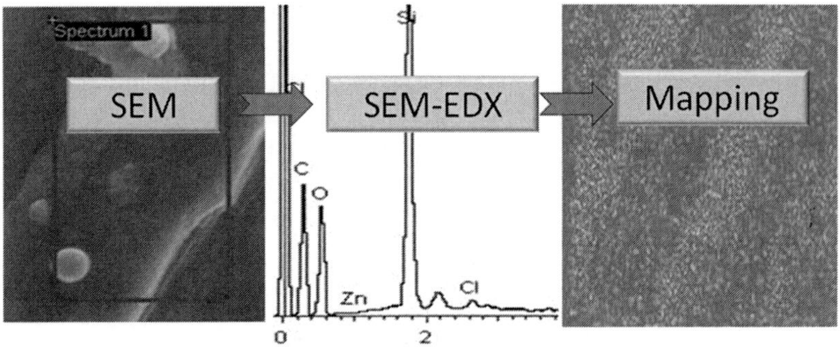

Figure 2.3[2]**. A**) SEM microphotograph of ZnO nanoparticle and homogenous coating layer on cellulose materials with specified area used for EDX investigation, The purple square is the area that was scanned for mapping (C); **B**) Results of the SEM-EDX investigation with the proof that the cellulose material was successfully modified with the ZnO coating, **C**) SEM-EDX mapping was additionally performed on a specified area of the cellulose material in order to detect ZnO nanoparticles (gray dots on the figure) showing a homogenous coating, as proof of successful modification. Magnification of C was 1000 times

In order to systematically analyse and interpret the results obtained from the experimental study, a mathematical model was developed. This model encapsulates the relationship between the response (outcome) of the experiment and the various parameters that were investigated. Specifically, the concentrations of reagents (GLYMO, HCl, and ZnO nanoparticles), ultrasonic irradiation power, and time were selected as the independent variables in this investigation.

Interactions among these independent variables were graphically presented in Figure 2.4.

This figure comprises a set of 3D response surface plots, each corresponding to one of the investigated parameters. The effects of ultrasonic power are delineated with respect to various factors, namely:

a) The concentration of GLYMO
b) The concentration of HCl

c) The concentration of ZnO nanoparticles
d) The time of the modification process

Indeed, the creation of these detailed 3D response surface plots was a carefully orchestrated process, utilizing specialized software such as State Ease. These plots serve a critical purpose: they provide a visual depiction that sheds light on the intricate correlations and interactions that exist among the specific independent variables under scrutiny. By examining these plots, researchers gain valuable insights into the complex relationships and synergies between the investigated parameters.

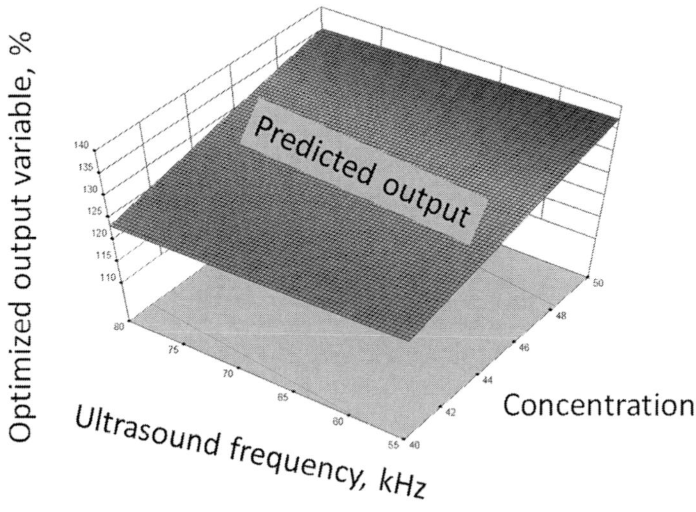

Figure 2.4. Three-dimensional response surface plots for investigating parameters: a) effects of the ultrasonic irradiation

This comprehensive perspective fosters a deeper understanding of how these variables collectively shape and influence the experimental outcomes. Essentially, the plots act as a graphical representation of the multifaceted dynamics at play within the experimental system. Furthermore, this approach has far-reaching implications. The interpretation of these plots empowers researchers to formulate well-grounded hypotheses and strategic approaches for optimizing the modification process. With a clearer comprehension of how changes in one parameter might impact others, researchers can fine-tune their experimental setup to achieve desired outcomes more effectively. In essence, these response surface plots become a visual tool that enhances the researcher's ability to navigate the complex landscape of experimental variables, ultimately driving progress and innovation in the field.

Figure 2.4 serves as an informative visualization, highlighting key trends and insights derived from the experimental results. Notably, the graph reveals that optimal outcomes are achieved when precursor GLYMO is present in higher concentrations, while HCl acid concentrations are kept lower. This observation underscores the delicate balance and synergy among the parameters. Moreover, the graph illuminates a noteworthy trend where lower concentrations of ZnO, coupled with higher ultrasound power and shorter time intervals, result in the heightened loading of nanoparticles onto the cellulose material. Conversely, an extended duration of sonication and greater power yield less effective nanoparticle loading. This intriguing phenomenon can be elucidated through a hypothesis that centers on the limited surface area available for nanoparticle interaction on the cellulose material [41]. The behavior of aggregated nanoparticles during sonication also plays a crucial role. The vigorous action of ultrasonic waves can lead to the collapse of bubbles, which, in turn, can dislodge aggregated nanoparticles from the cellulose surface. Additionally, smaller nanoparticles exhibit a propensity to permeate the material and adhere more firmly, resulting in increased aggregation during prolonged sonication. The eventual outcome is the removal of nanoparticle aggregates. This intricate interplay underscores the dynamic process through which nanoparticles are introduced to the cellulose material and distributed on its surface.

The loading of nanoparticles is influenced by a combination of nanoparticle concentration and sonication time. This revelation further underscores the multifaceted nature of the modification process and the interconnectedness of the parameters that influence the final outcome [41]. In essence, Figure 2.4 and the associated findings provide valuable insights that guide the understanding and optimization of the modification process, facilitating more informed decision-making and effective experimental design.

A pivotal indicator of an effective relaxation phenomenon is a high recovery angle value. This parameter assumes particular significance in the context of medical textiles, as it directly influences the material's comfort and softness when in contact with the skin. Given that the primary objective of surface modification on cellulosic materials was to render them suitable for use in medical textiles, the maximization of the recovery angle emerged as a central goal for optimization.

In pursuit of this objective, the modified cellulosic materials resulting from the 26 preliminary experiments underwent rigorous testing for their recovery angles. The evaluation followed the guidelines outlined in the EN ISO 22313: 2008 standard. By systematically assessing the recovery angles of these modified materials, researchers gained valuable insights into their potential comfort and softness attributes. This approach serves as a critical step in determining the suitability of these materials for medical textile applications, where user comfort and skin interaction are paramount concerns. Table 2.2 shows results that are recalculated as mean values from $n = 3$ experiments.

The obtained model is following:

"Recovery angle" = 108.92 + 0.34c(GLYMO (mol/dm-3)) − 0.018c(HCl(mol/dm-3)) + 72.28(m/g(ZnO)) + 0.19(Ultrasound power/Hz) – 0.03 (time/min) (2)

In order to assess the potential applicability of the developed model in predicting responses for the investigated parameters and optimizing the cellulose modification process, a thorough comparison was conducted between predicted values from the model and the actual experimental results. This comparison serves as a crucial step in evaluating the reliability and accuracy of the mathematical model. By juxtaposing the predicted outcomes with the real-world experimental data, researchers can gauge the model's effectiveness in capturing the intricate relationships and dynamics within the modification process. The degree of agreement or deviation between predicted and actual values provides valuable insights into the model's predictive power. This validation process is fundamental for establishing the model's credibility and potential utility in guiding future experimentation and optimization efforts. A strong alignment between predicted and experimental values suggests that the model holds promise for effectively predicting responses and optimizing the cellulose modification process. On the other hand, any disparities between predictions and actual results may necessitate further refinement or adjustment of the model to enhance its accuracy and reliability. The results are presented in Table 2.2.

Ž

Table 2.2. Comparison of predicted and actual values of recovery angles[2].

Predicted Recovery Angle	Actual Recovery Angle
135.7	135.8

The prediction of optimal parameter values for the cellulose modification process resulted in the following recommendations: 50 mL of GLYMO, m(ZnO) = 0.071 g, 50 mL of HCl (catalyzer) at a concentration of 0.1 mol/L, and ultrasonic irradiation at 80 kHz for a duration of 30.5 minutes. These predicted values were subsequently subjected to experimental verification, and the obtained results were then compared with the predicted values (as detailed in Table 2.2). The comparison between the predicted and experimentally obtained values is a critical step in validating the model's accuracy and reliability.

Remarkably, the relative error between the calculated and predicted values exhibited minuscule discrepancies, ranging from 0.007% to 0.670%. Additionally, the coefficient of variation (CV%), which reflects the variability of the selected model, demonstrated consistently low values. This outcome signifies an exceptional level of model precision and underscores the high reliability of the experimental outcomes. Based on this robust validation, the optimal combination of parameters was embraced for the formulation of the antibacterial coating. This optimal formulation was subsequently employed in the preparation of the coating to be tested for its antibacterial efficacy. With the optimal concentration of ZnO nanoparticles in place, rigorous testing was conducted to assess the zones of inhibition of bacterial growth and the minimum inhibitory concentrations (MICs) for the target bacteria, namely E. coli and S. aureus.

The results shown in Table 2.3 reveal stronger antibacterial activity against *S. aureus* compared to *E. coli* in both performed assays (Z.I. 37 mm vs. 24 mm and MIC 0.03 ppm vs. MIC 0.76 ppm, respectively) [42]. Indeed, the holistic strategy detailed in this study encapsulates a well-structured and methodical expedition toward achieving optimized modification processes and capitalizing on their potential to develop impactful antibacterial coatings tailored for medical applications.

This multifaceted approach begins with the prediction of optimal parameter values, leveraging a mathematical model that encapsulates the intricate relationships among various parameters. This predictive phase is followed by the crucial step of experimental validation, where the predicted values are put to the test in real-world scenarios. The remarkably low relative error and coefficient of variation observed during this validation underscore the model's accuracy and reliability.

With validated parameters in hand, the journey culminates in the formulation and creation of antibacterial coatings, meticulously designed to combat bacterial growth. Rigorous testing, including assessments of zones of inhibition and minimum inhibitory concentrations, demonstrates the tangible effectiveness of the modified materials.

By traversing through this comprehensive approach—from prediction to experimental validation and, finally, to antibacterial testing—researchers not only optimize the modification process but also unlock the potential for generating antimicrobial coatings with significant implications for medical applications. This iterative journey exemplifies the power of scientific inquiry and systematic exploration, ultimately driving innovation and progress in the realm of functional material development for medical and healthcare domains.

Table 2.3. Antibacterial activity of colloidal ZnO nanoparticles[2].

Microorganism	Diffusion (Z.I., mm)	Dillution (MIC)
S. aureus	37	0.03
E. coli	24	0.76

Furthermore, the efficacy of ZnO nanoparticles was scrutinized against two distinct strains of Staphylococcus aureus—Methicillin-Sensitive Staphylococcus aureus (MSSA) and Methicillin-Resistant Staphylococcus aureus (MRSA). The results revealed compellingly low Minimum Inhibitory Concentration (MIC) values, underscoring the potent antimicrobial potential of ZnO nanoparticles. For MRSA, the MIC value stood at a mere 3.28 ± 0.55 ppm, a testament to the nanoparticles' remarkable antimicrobial activity against this antibiotic-resistant strain. Even more strikingly, the MIC value for the S. aureus ATCC strain was an astonishingly low 0.03 ± 0.00 ppm, reinforcing the remarkable antimicrobial prowess of ZnO nanoparticles.

These findings serve as a compelling foundation for further exploration of ZnO nanoparticles in the realm of antimicrobial coatings. The exceptionally low MIC values lend strong support to the potential application of these nanoparticles in combating bacterial growth and infection. Moreover, the study extended its focus to coated cellulose materials that incorporated not only nanosized ZnO particles (with a size of 100 nm) but also significantly smaller nanosized platinum particles (measuring 3 nm). This exploration expands the horizon of antimicrobial coatings, leveraging the synergistic effects of multiple nanoparticle types to enhance their overall antimicrobial activity.

In summary, the investigation into ZnO nanoparticles' activity against distinct strains of S. aureus, coupled with the examination of combined nanoparticle coatings, showcases their promising potential for advancing the field of antimicrobial materials and coatings, with far-reaching implications for healthcare and beyond are shown in Figures 2.5 and 2.6.

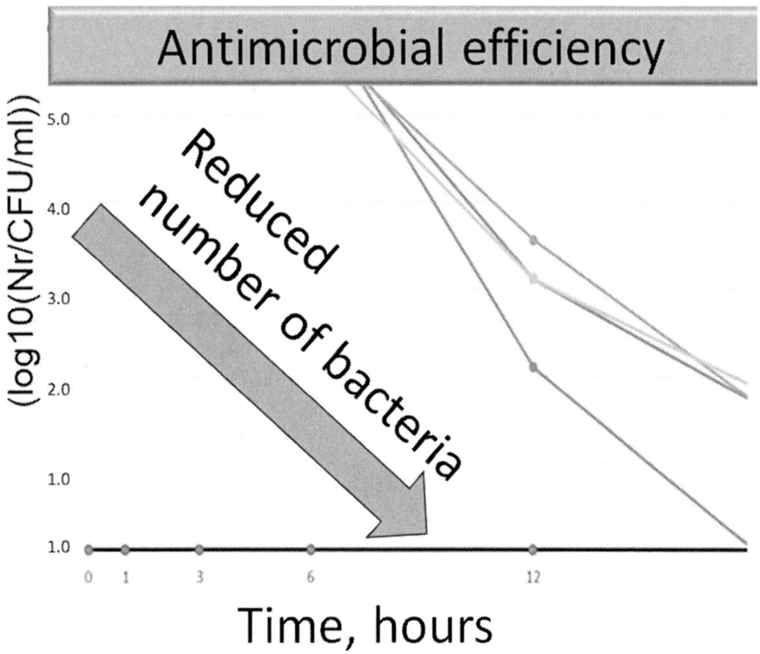

Figure 2.5. Graphic overview of reduced number of microorganisms on functionalized materials[2]

As can be seen from Figure 2.5, the investigation yielded a noteworthy observation: the onset of the antibacterial effect was notably pronounced after 6 hours of exposure to cellulose materials that had been modified with nanoparticles under ultrasonic irradiation. This distinct delay in antibacterial activity was in stark contrast to the controls, which encompassed untreated cellulose materials.

The outcome is visually depicted in Figure 2.5 and Figure 2.6, which succinctly illustrate the results of the antimicrobial experiments.

Remarkably, the cumulative effect of the modified materials was demonstrated by the complete elimination of viable bacteria across all investigated samples within a 24-hour timeframe. This outcome not only underscores the potency of the modified cellulose materials in combatting bacterial growth but also holds immense promise for future advancements in this scientific domain.

This breakthrough finding bears substantial implications, particularly in the context of preventing the spread of *Methicillin-Resistant Staphylococcus aureus (MRSA)*. While certain preventive measures, such as the use of disposable gloves, capes, and masks, can contribute to containment, they are not always a feasible solution. The urgency to counteract the propagation of antibiotic-resistant microorganisms necessitates the development of novel materials that exhibit strong antimicrobial activity. This success serves as a stepping stone, ushering in the potential for further pioneering research in this field. The prospect of developing advanced materials capable of combating antibiotic-resistant microorganisms could revolutionize infection control measures and pave the way for enhanced medical interventions. As such, this remarkable outcome not only addresses a pressing global health concern but also catalyzes a new era of innovation and progress in the realm of antimicrobial materials.

This chapter undertook a systematic exploration into the impact of various process parameters on the structure, morphology, and antimicrobial activity of coatings infused with zinc oxide nanoparticles. The parameters under scrutiny were thoughtfully manipulated across their designated ranges, involving ultrasonic irradiation power (ranging from 40 to 90 kHz), the concentration of reagents (encompassing nanoparticles, precursor, and acids), and the duration of sonication (ranging from 15 to 72 minutes).

The outcomes derived from this investigation unveiled an intricate interplay among the parameters and their effects on the presence and distribution of nanoparticles on the cellulose material. Notably, the concentration of reagents, ultrasonic irradiation power, and the duration of sonication emerged as pivotal determinants influencing the number of nanoparticles integrated into the cellulose material. Conversely, the impact of other parameters appeared to be comparatively less significant. Furthermore, the exploration into ultrasonic irradiation's influence highlighted an intriguing observation. Both ultrasonic irradiation power and duration demonstrated a synergistic role in shaping the modification process of the cellulose layer, particularly at lower temperatures. This synergistic interaction, when combined with varying reagent concentrations, exhibited a complex and multifaceted interdependence that manifested in the alteration of the cellulose material's properties.

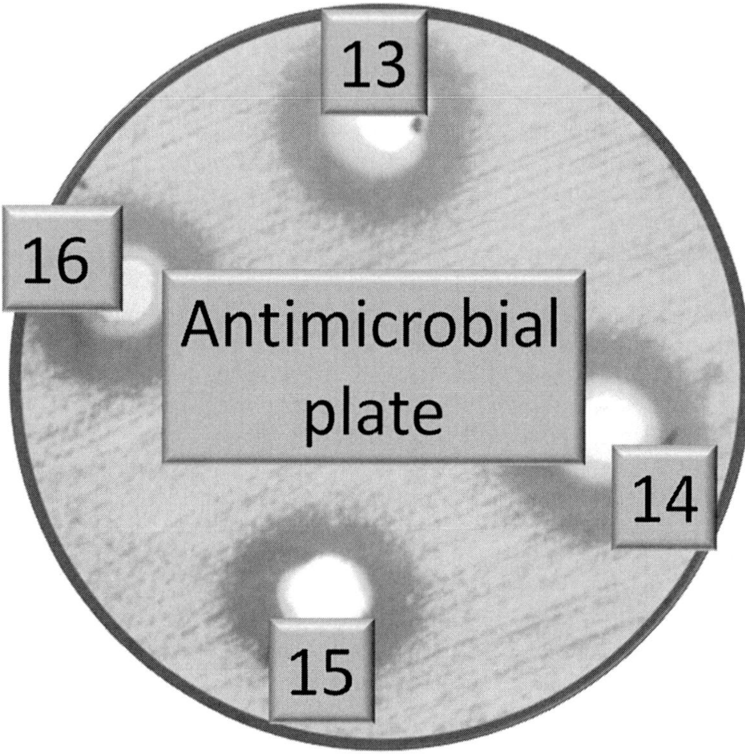

Figure 2.6. The plate after antimicrobial tests shows potent antimicrobial activity against tested microorganisms

In summation, this chapter's comprehensive analysis has significantly expanded our understanding of how specific process parameters orchestrate the modification of cellulose materials with zinc oxide nanoparticles. The intricate relationships unveiled in this study provide a solid foundation for further exploration and optimization, with the potential to open new avenues for the development of innovative antimicrobial coatings and functional materials.

Zinc oxide (ZnO) nanoparticles were ingeniously chemically tethered to the surface of cellulose through the meticulous sol-gel process, thereby yielding an antibacterial functionalized material. The application of ZnO nanoparticles was accomplished with remarkable efficiency at ambient pressure and low temperatures, resulting in the formation of a uniform and homogenous coating. An intriguing insight emerged from the study: a lengthened period of sonication and higher ultrasonic power engendered a diminishing efficacy in loading nanoparticles onto the cellulose material.

This observation underscored the pivotal role of ultrasonic irradiation as a critical parameter essential for achieving a consistent, antimicrobial, and efficacious surface. The conjunction of scanning electron microscope (SEM) images and Fourier transform infrared (FTIR) spectra provided compelling evidence of new chemical bonds forming and the successful adhesion of ZnO nanoparticles onto the material's surface. Subsequent antibacterial assays corroborated the material's potent antimicrobial attributes.

Statistical analyses conducted further unveiled the dependence of nanoparticle quantity on cellulose material upon the concentration of reagents, ultrasonic irradiation power, and sonication duration. The derived model highlighted optimal conditions for crafting an antimicrobial material endowed with exceptional flexibility. These conditions hinged upon specific reagent concentrations (ZnO at 0.071 g and HCl at 0.1 M) as well as ultrasonic irradiation at 80 kHz. Impressively, the model's predictions closely aligned with experimental outcomes, attesting to a remarkably low relative error spanning from 0.007% to 0.670%. In essence, ultrasonic irradiation, encompassing power and duration, played a harmonizing role alongside reagent concentration in the cellulose modification process at lower temperatures. This multi-dimensional interplay was deftly explored and understood through meticulous experimentation and data analysis. The cumulative findings underscore the profound significance of ultrasonic irradiation and its interconnected dynamics in tailoring antimicrobial cellulose surfaces, fostering a realm of possibilities for innovative applications in various domains.

References

1. World Health Organization. Antimicrobial Resistance Global Report on Surveillance 2014. Available online: https//www.who.int/drugresistance/documents/surveillancereport/en/(accessed on January 2020).
2. van Hal, S.J.; Jensen, S.O.; Vaska, V.L.; Espedido, B.A.; Paterson, D.L.; Gosbell, I.B. Predictors of mortality in Staphylococcus aureus Bacteremia. *Clin. Microbiol. Rev.* **2012**, *25*, 362–386.
3. Seil, J.T.; Webster, T.J. Antimicrobial applications of nanotechnology methods and literature. *Int. J. Nanomed.* **2012**, *7*, 2767–2781.
4. Azam, A.; Ahmed, A.S.; Oves, M.; Khan, M.S.; Habib, S.S.; Memic, A. Antimicrobial activity of metal oxide nanoparticles against Gram-

positive and Gram-negative bacteria a comparative study. *Int. J. Nanomed.* **2011**, *7*, 6003–6009.
5. Padmavathy, N.; Vijayaraghavan, R. Enhanced bioactivity of ZnO nanoparticles-an antimicrobial study. *Sci. Technol. Adv. Mater.* **2008**, *9*, 035004.
6. Saraf, R. Cost effective and monodispersed zinc oxide nanoparticles synthesis. *Int. J. Adv. Appl. Sci.* **2013**, *2*, 85–88.
7. Liu, Q.; Zhang, M.; Fang Zx Rong, X.H. Effect of homogenization and ultrasonication on the physical properties of insoluble wheat bran fibres. *J. Sci. Food Agric.* **2014**, *94*, 2547–2554.
8. Beyth, N.; Houri-Haddad, Y.; Domb, A.; Khan, W.; Hazan, R. Alternative Antimicrobial Approach Nano-Antimicrobial Materials. *Complement. Altern. Med.* **2015**, *2015*, 246012.
9. Dizaj, S.M.; Lotpoura, F.; Barzegar-Jalali, M.; Zarrintana, M.H.; Adibkiab, K. Antimicrobial activity of the metals and metal oxide nanoparticles. *Mater. Sci. Eng. C* **2014**, *44*, 278–284.
10. Emami-Karvani, Z.; Chehrazi, P. Antibacterial activity of ZnO nanoparticle on gram-positive bacteria. *Afr. J. Microbiol. Res.* **2011**, *5*, 1368–1373.
11. Rasmussen, J.W.; Martinez, E.; Louka, P.; Wingett, D.G. Zinc oxide nanoparticles for selective destruction of tumor cells and potential for drug delivery applications. *Expert Opin. Drug Deliv.* **2010**, *7*, 1063–1077.
12. Brayner, R.; Ferrari-Iliou, R.; Brivois, N.; Djediat, S.; Benedetti, M.F.; Fievet, F. Toxicological impact studies based on Escherichia coli bacteria in ultrafine ZnO nanoparticles colloidal medium. *Nano Lett.* **2006**, *6*, 866–870.
13. Jones, N.; Ray, B.; Ranjit, K.T.; Manna, A.C. Antibacterial activity of ZnO nanoparticle suspensions on a broad spectrum of microorganisms. *FEMS Microbiol. Lett.* **2008**, *279*, 71–76.
14. Jalal, R.; Goharshadi, E.K.; Abareshi, M.; Moosavi, M.; Yousefi, A.; Nancarrow, P. ZnO nanofluids: Green synthesis, characterization. *Mater. Chem. Phys.* **2008**, *121*, 198–201.
15. Raghupathi, K.R.; Koodali, R.T.; Manna, A.C. Size-dependent bacterial growth inhibition and mechanism of antibacterial activity of zinc oxide nanoparticles. *Langmuir* **2011**, *27*, 4020–4028.
16. Xie, Y.; He, Y.; Irwin, P.L.; Jin, T.; Shi, X. Combined Fluxomics and Transcriptomics Analysis of Glucose Catabolism via a Partially Cyclic Pentose Phosphate Pathway in *Gluconobacter oxydans* 621H. *Appl. Environ. Microbiol.* **2011**, *77*, 2325–2331.

17. Fan, Z.; Lu, J.G. Zinc oxide nanostructures: Synthesis and properties. *J. Nanosci. Nanotechnol.* **2005**, *5*, 1561–1573.
18. Song, Z.; Kelf, T.A.; Sanchez, W.H.; Roberts, M.S.; Ricka, J.; Frenz, M.; Zvyagin, A.V. Characterization of optical properties of ZnO nanoparticles for quantitative imaging of transdermal transport. *Biomed. Opt. Express* **2011**, *2*, 3321–3333.
19. Abramova, A.V.; Abramova, V.O.; Bayazitova, V.M.; Voitova, Y.; Straumal, E.A.; Lermontov, S.A.; Cherdyntseva, T.A.; Braeutigam, P.; Weiße, M.; Günther, K. A sol-gel method for applying nanosized antibacterial particles to the surfaceof textile materials in an ultrasonic field. *Ultrason. Sonochem.* **2020**, *60*, 104788.
20. Akhavan, F.; Majid Montazer, S. In situ sonosynthesis of nano TiO2 on cotton fabric. *Ultrason. Sonochem.* **2014**, *21*, 681–691.
21. Behzadnia, A.; Montazer, M.; MahmoudiRad, M. In situ photo sonosynthesis and characterize nonmetal/metal dual doped honeycomb-like ZnO nanocomposites on wool fabric. *Ultrason. Sonochem.* **2015**, *27*, 200–209.
22. Ahmadizadegan, H.; Esmaielzadeha, S.; Ranjbara, M.; Marzban, Z.; Ghavas, F. Synthesis and characterization of polyester bionanocomposite membrane with ultrasonic irradiation process for gas permeation and antibacterial activity. *Ultrason. Sonochem.* **2018**, *41*, 538–550.
23. Ghayempour, S.; Montazer, M. Ultrasound irradiation based in-situ synthesis of star-like Tragacanth gum/zinc oxide nanoparticles on cotton fabric. *Ultrason. Sonochem.* **2017**, *34*, 458–465.
24. Khan, M.F.; Ansari, A.H.; Hameedullah, M.; Ahmad, E.; Husain, F.M.; Zia, Q.; Baig, U.; Zaheer, M.R.; Alam, M.M.; Khan, A.M.; et al. Sol-gel synthesis of thorn-like ZnO nanoparticles endorsing mechanical stirring effect and their antimicrobial activities Potential role as nano-antibiotics. *Nat. Sci. Rep.* **2016**, *6*, 27689, doi10.1038/srep27689.
25. Barata, C.; Varo, I.; Navarro, J.C.; Arun, S.; Porte, C. Antioxidant enzyme activities and lipid peroxidation in the freshwater cladoceran Daphnia magna exposed to redox cycling compounds. *Toxicol. Pharmacol.* **2005**, *140*, 175–186.
26. Liu, J.; Fan, D.; Wang, L.; Shi, L.; Ding, J.; Chen, Y.; Shen, S. Effects of ZnO, CuO, Au, and TiO2 nanoparticles on *Daphnia magna* and early life stages of *zebrafish danio rerio* Env. Protect. Eng. 2014, 40, 139–1491.
27. Seabra, A.B.; Durán, N. Nanotoxicology of Metal Oxide Nanoparticles. *Metals* **2015**, *5*, 934–975.

28. Wang, N.; Magdassi, S.; Madnler, D.; Long, Y. Simple sol-gel process and one-step annealing of vanadium dioxide thin films: Synthesis and thermochromic properties. *Thin Solid Film.* **2013**, *534*, 594–598.
29. Yadav, A.; Prasad, V.; Kathe, A.A.; Raj, S.; Yadav, D.; Sundaramoorthy, C.; Vigneshwaran, N. Functional finishing in cotton fabrics using zinc oxide nanoparticles. *Bull. Mater. Sci.* **2006**, *29*, 641–645.
30. Vigneshwaran, N.; Kumar, S.; Kathe, A.A.; Varadarajan, P.V.; Prasad, V. Functional finishing of cotton fabrics using zinc oxide soluble starch nanocomposites. *Nanotechnology* **2006**, *17*, 5087–5095.
31. Rezić, I. Cellulosic fibers-biosorptive materials and indicators of heavy metals pollution. *Microchem. J.* **2013**, *107*, 63–69.
32. Council of Europe.; *European Pharmacopoeia* Commission, *European Pharmacopoeia*, 5th ed.; Council of Europe: Strasbourg, France, 2005; pp. 188–191.
33. European Committee for Antimicrobial Susceptibility Testing (EUCAST) of the European Society for Clinical Microbiology and Infectious Diseases (ESCMID). EUCAST Discussion Document E.Def.5.1. *Clin. Microbiol. Infec.* **2003**, *9*, 1–7.
34. Peran, J.; Ercegović Ražić, S.; Kosalec, I.; Ziberi, F. Antimicrobial Effectiveness of Cellulose based Fabrics treated with Silver Nitrate Solution using Plasma Processes.*Tekstilec* **2017**, *60*, 247–253.
35. Rezić, I. Optimization of ultrasonic extraction of 23 elements from cotton. *Ultrason. Sonochem.* **2009**, *16*, 63–69.
36. Rolich, T.; Rezić, I.; Ćurković, L. Estimation of Steel Guitar Strings Corrosion by Artificial Neural Network. *Corr. Sci.* **2010**, *52*, 996–1002.
37. Rezić, I.; Steffan, I. ICP-OES determination of metals present in textile materials. *Microchem. J.* **2007**, *85*, 46–51.
38. Rezić, I.; Ćurković, L.; Ujević, M. Simple methods for characterization of metals in historical textile threads. *Talanta* **2010**, *82*, 237–244.
39. Rezić, I.; Špehar, M.; Jakovljević, S. Characterization of Ag and Au nanolayers on Cu alloys by TLC, SEM-EDS, and ICP-OES. *Mater. Corr.* **2017**, *68*, 560–565.
40. Rezić, I.; Zeiner, M.; Steffan, I. Determination of 28 selected elements in textiles by axially viewed inductively coupled plasma optical emission spectrometry. *Talanta* **2011**, *83*, 865–871.
41. Reza Mahdavi, S.; Talesh, T.A. The effect of ultrasonic irradiation on the structure, morphology and photocatalytic performance of ZnO nanoparticles by sol-gel method. *Ultrason. Sonochem.* **2017**, *39*, 504–510.

42. Pokrovac, I. diploma thesis, mentors Rezić I. and Kosalec I., Antimicrobial effect of colloidal nanoparticles of metals and metal oxides on MSSA and MRSA, University of Zagreb, Faculty of Phamacy and Biochemistry, 2018

CHAPTER THREE

HYDROFOBIC SUPERTOOLS[1]

Introduction

Polymer materials hold significant potential for functionalization through diverse surface treatments. Among these, the application of nanoparticles in coatings has demonstrated remarkable success in conferring excellent antimicrobial properties. Notably, augmenting these properties can be achieved through hydrophobic surface modification. This chapter sets forth a comprehensive objective: to delineate a method for fine-tuning process parameters to achieve exceptional hydrophobicity in polymer surfaces. This pursuit is underpinned by the adept utilization of a Design of Experiment (DoE) statistical methodology. By harnessing this approach, the intricacies of the process are modeled and optimized across six crucial processing parameters. The integration of response surface methodology, coupled with a center composite design, forms the bedrock of this endeavor. An essential facet entails subjecting the achieved results to the ANOVA (Analysis of Variance) test, a statistical analysis that serves as a vital gauge for the significance of all variables involved. In summation, this chapter offers a comprehensive exposé on the utilization of Design of Experiment as a potent tool for optimizing parameters that play a pivotal role in shaping hydrophobicity and surface functionalization. By navigating the intricate interplay of variables, this methodology affords an avenue for enhancing polymer surfaces' hydrophobic properties, thereby unlocking novel possibilities in diverse applications across a myriad of industries.

Hydrophobic finishing stands as a cornerstone within the textile industry, embodying one of its paramount processes. This crucial treatment imparts a distinctive trait to textile materials, endowing them with the ability to repel water, oil, and dry dirt. The profound significance of this finishing prowess reverberates across diverse domains, ranging from clothing and sportswear to military, medical, and technical textiles. [**1**].

---

[1] Rezić I., Kiš A., Design of Experiment Approach to Optimize Hydrophobic Fabric Treatments, P*olymers* 2020, *12*(9), 2131; https://doi.org/10.3390/polym12092131

The virtues of this hydrophobic finishing are manifold and far-reaching. By instilling textiles with the capability to shun water, these materials gain a valuable shield against moisture infiltration. In the realm of clothing, this translates to garments that remain impervious to rain, thereby ensuring wearer comfort and longevity. Sporting apparel benefits from extended use even in inclement weather conditions, while military uniforms gain an edge in the field by keeping moisture at bay.

Moreover, the medical and healthcare sector gains a distinct advantage through hydrophobic textiles, which can effectively repel fluids and contaminants. This property proves instrumental in maintaining hygiene and preventing the spread of pathogens, a critical consideration within healthcare settings. Technical textiles, underpinned by hydrophobic finishing, find application across a spectrum of industries, contributing to enhanced durability, resilience, and efficiency in diverse contexts.

In essence, the process of hydrophobic finishing holds a transformative potential that resonates across a multitude of sectors, ushering in enhanced functionality, extended longevity, and heightened versatility for textile materials. This pivotal procedure assumes a pioneering role within the ongoing evolution and innovation of the textile industry, deftly addressing a diverse array of needs and paving the path for future advancements.

Polymer materials, too, emerge as a canvas for remarkable transformation, acquiring the ability to combat resistant microorganisms through a spectrum of surface treatments. Notably, the incorporation of nanoparticles within surface coatings yields exceptional antimicrobial properties, underscoring the potential for groundbreaking advancements in material functionality.

Moreover, the augmentation of antimicrobial attributes can be further propelled by additional surface modifications that confer outstanding hydrophobic properties. This dual enhancement, where antimicrobial potency converges with exceptional water-repellent characteristics, unveils a realm of possibilities for creating textiles that are not only resistant to staining but also adept at repelling water, oil, and other compounds.

Delving into history, the utilization of water repellent materials traces a broad trajectory encompassing wax and resin compounds. However, contemporary applications have introduced perfluoroalkyl compounds (PFAS's) as a dominant player in stain-repellent finishes. These compounds stand unrivalled in their ability to simultaneously repel water, oil, dirt, and various other staining agents.

In summary, the textile industry's journey is intertwined with the ingenious utilization of hydrophobic finishing and the functionalization of polymer materials. These pursuits, powered by cutting-edge technologies and innovations, converge to shape a dynamic landscape marked by exceptional antimicrobial, hydrophobic, and staining-repellent properties. Through these endeavours, the industry continues to surge forward, meeting evolving challenges with unwavering ingenuity and opening avenues for transformative progress. [**3**].

Indeed, the pursuit of enhancing repellent properties in textile materials yields a cascade of positive effects that extend far beyond water and stain resistance. This concerted effort brings forth a plethora of improvements across various fabric properties, culminating in a comprehensive enhancement of material performance. One of the notable gains arises in the realm of chemical resistance. By fortifying the fabric with enhanced repellent properties, textiles exhibit heightened resilience against acids, bases, and an array of other chemicals. This newfound robustness equips the textiles to withstand exposure to potentially damaging substances, thereby expanding their utility across diverse applications. The impact extends to drying kinetics as well. Fabrics endowed with augmented repellent capabilities tend to dry more rapidly. This accelerated drying time not only contributes to user comfort by minimizing the duration of dampness but also holds potential benefits in specialized contexts where rapid moisture evaporation is imperative. Furthermore, the pursuit of enhanced repellent properties synergistically contributes to better durable press properties. The propensity of the fabric to retain its shape and resist wrinkling is notably improved. This yields textiles that maintain a well-groomed appearance even after extended periods of wear, further elevating their durability and longevity. In summation, the strategic elevation of repellent properties in textile materials cascades into a comprehensive enhancement of various fabric attributes. This holistic approach, encompassing chemical resistance, drying efficiency, and durable press properties, amplifies the material's overall performance and underscores the multifaceted benefits derived from a singular focus on repellent enhancements. As a result, the textile industry stands poised to offer products that not only resist stains and moisture but also excel across a spectrum of practical and functional dimensions. [**4**].

> Fluorocarbons are synthetically produced organic chemicals in which all hydrogen atoms are replaced by fluorine containing a perfluoroalkyl residue (**Figure 3.1**) [**1**]. Those chemicals exhibit a significant reduction in surface tension (due to their incompatibility with water and oil), and outstanding stability (both chemical and thermal) [**3**].

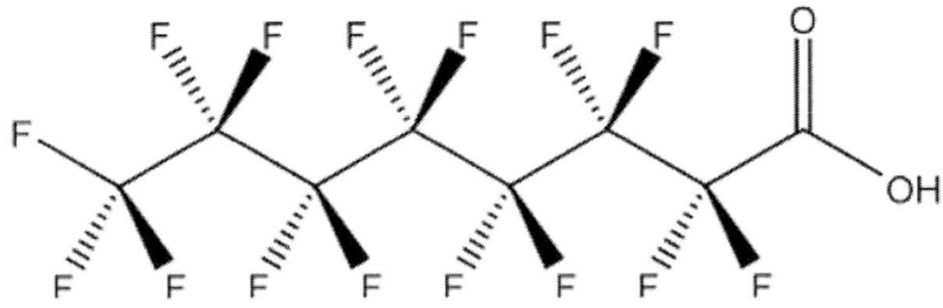

Figure 3.1. Perfluoro octane alcohol: $F_3C–CF_2–CF_2–CF_2–CF_2–CF_2–CF_2–CF_2–CF_2–CH_2–CH_2–OH$ [**3**].

Fluorocarbons, particularly certain types of perfluoroalkyl and polyfluoroalkyl substances (PFAS), have been associated with potential health and environmental concerns. These compounds, commonly used in various industrial applications including stain and water repellent finishes for textiles, have been found to persist in the environment and have been detected in water sources, soil, and even in the human body.

Research has indicated that some PFAS compounds can accumulate in living organisms and have been linked to adverse health effects, including potential developmental, reproductive, and immune system impacts. Due to these concerns, there has been increasing attention on regulating and reducing the use of certain fluorocarbons and PFAS compounds in consumer products and industrial processes.

It's important to note that there are various types of fluorocarbons with differing properties and potential impacts. The specific health and environmental risks associated with any given fluorocarbon compound may depend on factors such as its chemical structure, persistence, bioaccumulation potential, and how it is used. As our understanding of the potential risks of fluorocarbons continues to evolve, regulatory agencies and industries are working to better assess and manage the use of these compounds to ensure the safety of both human health and the environment. When considering the use of fluorocarbons, it's important to be aware of the potential risks and to make informed choices based on the available scientific knowledge and regulatory guidance.

Water repellence

The concept underlying repellence involves a reduction in free energy at the material surface [5]. In situations where the adhesive forces between the material and liquid drops surpass the internal cohesive interactions within the liquid, the drops will naturally disperse. Conversely, if adhesive interactions between the material and the liquid fall short of the internal cohesive interactions within the liquid, the liquid drops will remain undisturbed [6].

Numerous parameters wield influence over surface tension and, consequently, repellence, with chain length emerging as a noteworthy factor [3]. Existing literature highlights a rapid decrease in critical surface tension as chain length escalates from one to eight, followed by a subsequent decline [7]. However, the employment of 8 C-atom fluorocarbons ("C8") has raised environmental and health concerns, prompting the Croatian industry's adoption of C6 fluorocarbons starting from September 2020. These C6 variants, compliant with stringent regulations, will necessitate a heightened level of responsibility from industrial managers and process engineers. Their task extends beyond meeting rigorous ecological standards to also satisfying customer demands for super hydrophobic garments.

Cost-effective nanotechnology-based repellents have given rise to diverse treatments, yet refinement remains imperative due to the adverse impact of current products on comfort, particularly in hot and humid environments [8]. This impetus has led to a concerted drive towards enhancing not only repellence but also other protective attributes of garments. A spectrum of endeavors spans varied processing domains, encompassing fabric weave technology [9], coating innovation, surface nanocomposite modifications involving resins and nanoparticles [10], and the inventive integration of double-sided knitting featuring distinct fiber types [11].

The quest extends further to the realm of fabric functionality. Ambitious strides are being taken to achieve waterproof breathable fabrics [12], usher in super-hydrophobic and multi-responsive fabric composites boasting remarkable electro-photo-thermal effects [13], and not solely within textiles but also crossing over to composite insulators [14]. Moreover, the horizon beckons with the promise of intelligent electronic clothing systems [15] while concurrently exploring the domain of medical materials imbued with antibacterial prowess [16,17]. As these frontiers expand, the incorporation of membranes, coatings, fabrics, and other pivotal variables assumes a crucial role in the blueprinting of breathable garments [18].

A variety of parameters intricately influences material wear comfort, notably the porosity and strength of the micro-porous layer on textile material. This gamut encompasses facets such as crystallinity, stretching conditions, pressure, heat treatment specifics, reagent selection, and more [1].

To navigate this intricate web and unearth optimal conditions for multi-parameter processes, the Design of Experiment (DoE) statistical methodology emerges as a guiding beacon [19,20,21,22,23]. For instance, Moussa et al. harnessed a factorial experimental design to optimize the waterproof breathable attributes of samples [11], delving into the optimization of vital parameters. Coronado et al. ventured into a mixture design of experiments to assess the environmental implications of clay-based structural ceramics featuring hazardous metals [19], while Waha et al. orchestrated the process of biodegradation optimization through the Taguchi design of experiment [20]. In this fashion, the art and science of experimentation become powerful allies in the pursuit of unlocking the full potential of innovative textile treatments and garment designs.

Since the 1940s, synthetic compounds known as long chain fluor-chemicals, characterized by a minimum of eight perfluorinated carbon atoms, have found their way into an array of consumer and industrial products. These versatile substances have been integrated into firefighting foams, various surfaces, and even food contact paper. The consequence of their extensive utilization is their presence in the environment and within the human body. Regrettably, recent findings underscore the potential for adverse health consequences arising from sustained exposure to specific levels of certain long chain fluorochemicals [24]. Studies have illuminated the association between PFAS's (perfluoroalkyl substances) and reproductive toxicity, diminished newborn growth metrics, and elevated cholesterol levels in humans. Adding to the concern is the remarkable persistence and resistance to degradation exhibited by PFAS, rendering them a formidable global issue.

Looking ahead, projections paint a sobering picture: by 2050, the threat of infections caused by antibiotic-resistant bacteria could potentially surpass that of cancer in terms of mortality. Within Europe alone, a staggering toll of 25,000 deaths annually and a financial burden exceeding EUR 1.5 billion are attributed to resilient microorganisms. Among the roster of menacing bacterial infections, Staphylococcus aureus and its formidable variant Methicillin-resistant Staphylococcus aureus (MRSA), often dubbed "super-bacteria" or "golden staphylococci," stand as prominent adversaries.

The challenge posed by MRSA is compounded by its unyielding resistance to a broad spectrum of antibiotic-based penicillin drugs, notably the β-lactam antibiotics like methicillin, dicloxacillin, nafcillin, and oxacillin. Staphylococcus aureus, a gram-positive bacterium characterized by spherical forms, belongs to the S*taphylococcaceae* family and ranks among the most formidable global pathogens. Its prevalence ranges from 20 to 50 cases per 100,000 inhabitants annually, with mortality rates ranging from 10% to 30%, marking a concerning fatality outcome. Remarkably, this toll eclipses the combined deaths attributed to AIDS, tuberculosis, and viral hepatitis, underscoring the gravity of the challenge at hand.

This chapter endeavours to elucidate the evolution of a hydrophobic polymer surface, poised to serve as a prospective antimicrobial material. The core objective entails attaining remarkable hydrophobic attributes, meticulously honed through the optimization of textile functionalization process parameters. This intricate pursuit of optimization was meticulously orchestrated across six pivotal process variables, executed by harnessing the potent tool of Design of Experiment methodology.

> The goal of optimization was to find optimal conditions of the water vapor permeability and the resistance to water wetting. The analysis of water vapor permeability is related to the level of comfort at low physical activity but does not give the information about condensation on a textile surface.

The scope of this study encompassed a comprehensive analysis of three distinct textile material samples, meticulously tailored for potential application in military attire. These samples were meticulously fashioned from cotton and polyamide yarns, distinguished by varying weights of 190 g/m2, 220 g/m2, and 240 g/m2. An in-depth exploration of the mechanical attributes of these samples is thoughtfully detailed and succinctly summarized in Table 3.1.

Table 3.1. Mechanical properties of investigated samples.

Property of sample	Sample 1	Sample 2	Sample 3
Weight, g/m^2	190	220	240
Fabric Composition	50% Cardura (PA 6.6.)/50% cotton		

The textile finishing treatment also encompassed the integration of a distinctive dye - Bezathren Navy Blue GN vat dye, a creation of CHT hailing from Montlingen, Switzerland. Notably distinguished for its exceptional light, wet, and chlorine fastness attributes on cellulose fibers, this dye was harnessed to augment the textile modification process. Its application was facilitated in the form of a micro-disperse powder, ensuring ease of dispersion and seamless integration into the textile modification process.

The evaluation encompassed the examination of two distinct hydrophobic compounds: a fluorocarbon agent derived from C8 fluorochemicals, denoted as *Sevophob HFK–F,* and a fluorocarbon agent rooted in C6 fluorochemicals, known as T*ubiguard SCS-F. Sevophob HFK–*

F, crafted as a fluorocarbon resin is renowned for its efficacy in conferring permanent water, oil, and dirt repellence to surfaces. Likewise, *Tubiguard SCS-F*, a low-viscosity liquid dispersion produced by CHT, emerged as a contender in this hydrophobic exploration. Concentration ranges spanning from 35 to 70 g/L were examined for each compound.

The process employed for the transformation of the material into a hydrophobic textile involved a meticulous textile finishing treatment, entailing the pad impregnation of fabric and dyeing, coupled with the application of specialized finishing chemicals. This multifaceted procedure was methodically structured and executed in several key steps, elucidated as follows:

1. Pre-Treatment: The initial phase encompassed pre-treatment, designed to expunge impurities such as waste, oil, dry matter, and other contaminants, setting the foundation for subsequent modifications.
2. Dyeing: The fabric underwent a dyeing process, involving the infusion of color through immersion in a dye solution.
3. Finishing with Hydrophobic Agents: The ensuing step involved the integration of finishing chemicals, specifically two distinct types of fluorocarbon agents. This dual-pronged approach aimed to bestow the fabric with water and oil repellency, contributing to its hydrophobic attributes.

Notably, the latter two steps, encompassing dyeing and finishing experiments, were meticulously executed on a laboratory scale. This involved the utilization of specialized laboratory machinery designed for the pad impregnation process.

During this process, the fabric was guided through a solution containing the dye and chemicals via a submerged roller. As the fabric emerged from the bath, it underwent mechanical pressure between two cylinders, facilitating the removal of excess solution. This precise mechanical impregnation technique aimed to ensure an even distribution of the solution or chemical dispersion across the fabric, thereby achieving the desired hydrophobic modification.

> The pivotal factor governing both thermological and physiological comfort of textile materials is the process of moisture transport. This intricate mechanism involves the movement of moisture through a material, occurring in the dual forms of vapours or liquids. A critical parameter used to quantify this phenomenon is the water vapor permeability (WVP), which delineates the rate at which water vapor traverses a designated unit area. This rate is contingent upon the vapor pressure disparity between two distinct surfaces, all within predefined temperature and humidity parameters. In essence, WVP serves as a quantitative measure of the efficiency with which a textile material facilitates the transmission of water vapor, a fundamental attribute contributing to overall comfort. [**25**].

Water vapor permeability, (WVP) can be calculated as: $WVP = (G \times A \times \Delta p)/\mathrm{t}$ where Δp, (Pa) is the difference of partial pressure between two sides of material, G, (g)—weight change, t, (h)—time during which G occurred, and A, (m^2)—test area.

As per the ASTM E96 standard procedure, the evaluation entails the following steps: A circular sample is securely affixed onto a test cup, which is subsequently filled with distilled water. The prepared test cup, containing the sample, is positioned within a closely regulated environment. This controlled setting maintains an ambient temperature of 23.0 °C, coupled with a relative humidity of 100% within the confines of the cup and 50% outside it.

The underlying principle driving the assessment involves the interplay of concentration and pressure differentials. Within this controlled environment, vapor diffusion ensues through the textile material, originating from the cup and progressing into the external surroundings. This process is facilitated by the inherent forces arising from the disparities in concentration and pressure. The resultant measurement yields valuable insights into the water vapor permeability of the textile under examination. [**25**].

Subsequent to the hydrophobic modification, an evaluation of the modification's durability was conducted through a series of washing cycles. This durability testing encompassed a 5-cycle process, meticulously executed in accordance with the specifications delineated in the norm EN ISO 6330:2012. Specifically, the procedures outlined within this standard pertaining to domestic washing and drying of textiles were rigorously adhered to. The entire testing regimen was carried out at a temperature of 60 °C.

Concurrently, the water vapor permeability (WVP) of the modified textile material was assessed. This assessment hewed closely to the established guidelines stipulated by the ASTM E96 standard procedure. Within the context of this procedure, the movement of vapor was observed to transition from the interior to the exterior of a designated cup. The ASTM E96 standard procedure was conscientiously followed, affording a comprehensive understanding of the material's water vapor transmission properties. (**Figure 3.2**).

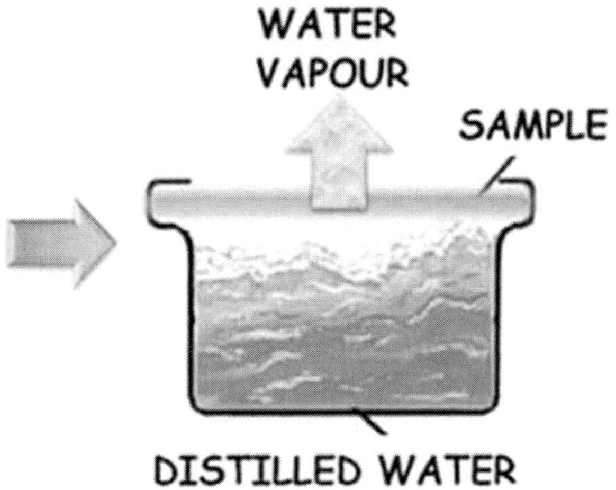

Figure 3.2. Schematic overview of test for vapor permeability by the ASTM E96 method.

However, it's important to acknowledge a limitation inherent in this methodology. The permeability measurements derived from this approach are influenced not solely by the material's intrinsic properties, but also by the thickness of the air layer in proximity to the textile surface. Recognizing this inherent constraint, a complementary set of experiments was undertaken to evaluate the material's resistance to surface wetting.

This assessment of resistance to surface wetting was meticulously conducted in strict accordance with the ISO 4920:2012 standard procedure. By adhering to this established protocol, a comprehensive understanding of the material's ability to resist surface wetting was obtained, thus providing a well-rounded characterization of its hydrophobic properties. [**26**].

This technique, as outlined by the ISO 4920:2012 standard procedure, entails the application of a spray test to evaluate a fabric's resistance to surface wetting by water. The process entails the controlled spraying of a predefined volume of distilled water onto a test specimen affixed to a ring, positioned at a specific 45° angle. The specimen's central point is deliberately situated at a designated distance beneath the spray nozzle. Subsequently, the spray rating is ascertained by juxtaposing the appearance of the test specimen against predetermined descriptive benchmarks.

The intricate data generated from these experiments underwent meticulous analysis, facilitated by the utilization of Design Expert Stat Ease software 9.1 (Minneapolis, MN, USA). To ensure robust statistical insights, a central composite design was judiciously selected as the modeling framework. This encompassed six key process parameters, each subjected to replicates, ultimately yielding a total of 42 meticulously orchestrated experiments. Through this methodical approach, a comprehensive and accurate depiction of the fabric's resistance to surface wetting was achieved.

The optimal parameter settings for six distinct independent variables were determined through the application of advanced algorithms within the *Design Expert State Ease* version 9.1 software (Minneapolis, MN, USA). These variables encompassed fabric weight, dye concentration, concentrations of the hydrophobic compounds *Sevophob HFK–F* and *Tubiguard SCS–F*, temperature, pressure, and the specific type of hydrophobic compound employed.

It is noteworthy that the critical surface tension of hydrophobic compounds exhibits a distinct trend, characterized by a rapid decline as the chain length increases from 1 to 8, followed by a subsequent decrease [7]. In industrial processes, fluorocarbons consisting of 8 carbon atoms were widely utilized due to their exceptional hydrophobic attributes. However, the undeniable adverse environmental and human health repercussions associated with these compounds have led to their prohibition. Consequently, this study undertook a systematic exploration and optimization of various treatments employing both C6 and C8 fluorocarbons, leveraging the manipulation of six distinct industrial process parameters.

> This statistical program DoE searches for an optimal combination of factor levels that simultaneously satisfies the requirements placed on each of the responses and factors.

Sevophob HFK–F and *Tubiquard SCS–F*, both fluor-based finishing compounds, were subject to thorough investigation in this research as potential hydrophobic agents for achieving robust and enduring finishes on military garments. Notably, *Sevophob HFK-F*, although more potent, contains eight carbon atoms in its structural composition, while *Tubiquard SCS-F* possesses only six carbon atoms.

To attain comparably satisfactory outcomes using an environmentally conscientious reagent, a comprehensive multi-parameter optimization strategy was undertaken through the application of Design of Experiment (DoE) methodology.

This approach encompassed the exploration of six distinct process parameters, specifically: military fabric weight (ranging from 190 to 240 g/m2), dye concentration (10 to 60 g/L), hydrophobic compound concentration (35 to 70 g/L), hydrophobic compound type (varying from six to eight carbon atoms), temperature (ranging from 150 to 170 °C), and pressure (from 1.0 to 2.0 bar).

The optimization process involved conducting 42 preliminary experiments wherein these six input process variables were systematically varied, all with the overarching objective of optimizing the hydrophobic characteristics of the garments while upholding the comfort of the materials when worn.

Traditional optimization protocols, characterized by the sequential alteration of one parameter at a time, often fall short in providing insights into the intricate interactions between process variables and their collective impact on the final outcome within an industrial setting. The application of Design of Experiment (DoE) statistical methodology offers a compelling solution to this challenge. It enables the study of the effects of process variables and their corresponding responses within a minimal number of preliminary experiments, thus yielding a more comprehensive understanding of the underlying dynamics of the industrial process. [**27**].

Design of Experiment

By employing Design of Experiments (DoE) grounded in the principles of Response Surface Methodology (RSM), facilitated through the State Ease software, an optimized combination of mix proportions was determined, effectively leading to a significant reduction in the total number of required experiments. The utilization of DoE within the RSM framework enables a more efficient and structured approach to parameter exploration and optimization. To ascertain the presence of a discernible relationship between the designated parameters and the respective response variables under investigation, a rigorous statistical analysis of the collected data was imperative. This analysis was conducted through a regression process, in accordance with the following equation:

$$x_i = (X_i - X_{xi})/\Delta X_i.$$

where x_i is the coded value of the independent variable i, X_i the natural value of the variable i, X_i^x the natural value of the variable i in the central point and ΔX_i is the value of the step change.

The response y is the estimation of the coefficients of a quadratic model, and it can be represented by equation within the central composite design:

$$y=\beta_0+\sum_{i=1}^{k} \beta_i x_i+\sum_{i=1}^{k} \beta_{ii}x^2_i+\sum_{i<j} \beta_{ii} x_i x_j+\varepsilon$$

where, y is the measured response, β_0 is the intercept term, β_i, β_{ii} and β_{ij} are the measures of the effects of variables x_i, $x_i x_j$ and x_{2i}, respectively. The central composite design was selected since this is one of the most efficient and popular classes of second order designs recommended in the literature [**19**]. A very important optimization step is the selection of parameters and their ranges to be studied, which was done based on previous analysis. The factors were studied in several levels, from low to high, as is presented in **Table 3.2**.

The worst result in the preliminary tests was recorded in the eighth experiment (with 1196 g/m^2 for water vapor permeability), for the hydrophobic compound with six C atoms.

Table 3.2. Experimental planning in Design of Experiment, central composite design, six parameters, 42 preliminary experiments, six input parameters and two output responses.[3]

Input parameters:			
Description	Title	Min.	Max.
FC-compound C6 levels	TUBIGUARD SCS-F	20 g/l	60 g/l
Auxiliarry for enhancing resistance to washing of resins	TUBICOAT FIXIERER FC	10 g/l	20 g/l
Accelerator	KOLLASOL CDO	0,1 g/l	0,3 g/l
Pressure of fular		1 bar	2 bar

Output parameters: Water repellence– before and after 5 machine cyclus at 60°C; Oil repellence - before and after 5 machine cyclus at 60°C; Designed experiments:					
Nr	Fabric	FC6	FIXIER	ACCELERATOR,	Pressure
1	310	40	15	0.3	1
2	220	20	10	0.3	1
3	220	32	10.5	0.23	1.665
4	220	48.3212	10	0.1	1
5	220	32	10.5	0.23	1.665
6	310	60	20	0.1	1
7	310	60	20	0.3	2
8	220	20	20	0.3	2
9	310	20	10	0.3	2
10	220	60	20	0.3	1
11	310	40.8	20	0.2	1.495
12	310	60	10	0.3	1
13	310	52.4	15.8735	0.17578	2
... (continues, see reference[3] for more details 1) ...					
42	220	44	17	0.3	1.6

The experimental design matrix consisted of 42 experiments, strategically structured using a central composite design encompassing three levels of factors. This comprehensive design matrix was employed to construct a quadratic model, aiming to capture and elucidate the intricate relationships within the observed response data. The graphical representation of the standard error of the design is illustrated in Figure 3.3, effectively portraying the variability of the predicted mean. Notably, a larger standard error signifies a reduced level of reliability in the estimations.

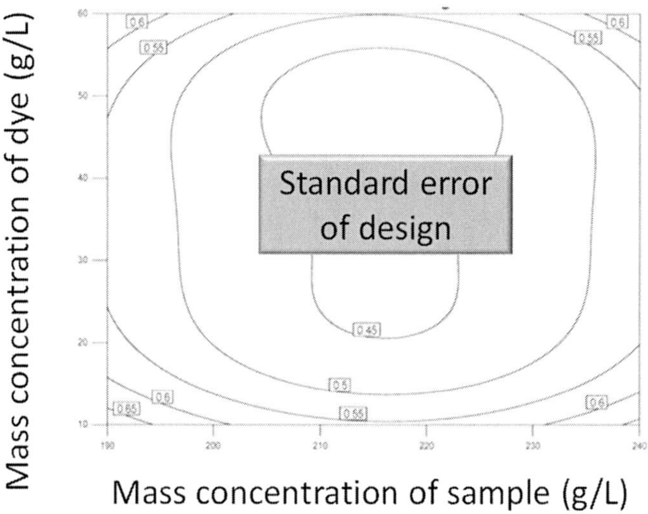

Figure 3.3. Standard error of design[3].

ANNOVA

The analysis of variance (ANOVA) was carried out to establish the significance of different parameters for the quadratic model. The quadratic model for the water vapor permeability in terms of coded factors is presented as:

$$\text{Water Repellency} = 87.41 - 1.19 \times A + 0.12 \times B + 0.49 \times C + 4.02 \times D - 0.20 \times E - 9.87 \times F + 0.15 \times AB + 0.33 \times AC + 3.81 \times AD - 3.96 \times AE - 2.23 \times AF - 1.64 \times BC - 6.21 \times BD - 0.012 \times BE + 3.56 \times BF - 0.34 \times CD - 1.21 \times CE + 0.048 \times CF - 0.91 \times DE + 2.89 \times DF + 0.49 \times EF + 3.07 \times B2 - 4.85 \times C2 - 1.14 \times D2 + 0.64 \times E2$$

where coded parameters are: A Fabric weight, B Dye concentration, C Hydrophobic auxiliary compounds concentration, D Temperature and E the Pressure.

The significance of parameters is established by assessing their p-values, with a threshold of 0.05 serving as the significance limit. In the context of this model, each parameter exhibited noteworthy significance, as indicated by their respective p-values of 0.0020, 0.0109, 0.0005, 0.0220, 0.0010, and 0.0001, corresponding to fabric weight, dye concentration, hydrophobic compound concentration, temperature, and pressure. The computed model F-value of 4.22 further substantiates the model's significance, attaining a 95% confidence level.

Furthermore, when analysing the p-value "p > F," a value below 0.0500 indicates the significance of model terms. In this study, the p-value was found to be 0.0022. The assessment of lack of fit, derived from experimental errors and residuals, yielded a "Lack of fit F-value" of 10.13, accompanied by a p-value of 0.0096, signifying significant lack of fit. Consequently, the proposed model for water vapor permeability is deemed valid and applicable within the scope of the current investigation. **Figure 3.4** compares experimental values with the predicted model.

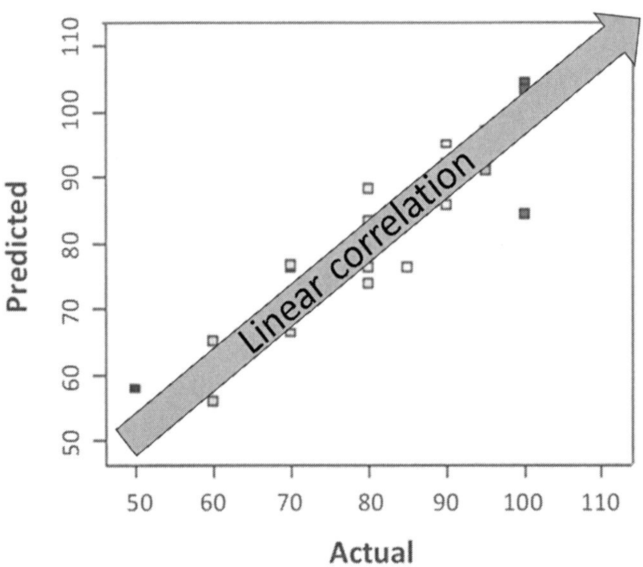

Figure 3.4. Plot of actual value and the value predicted by DoE

The Durbin–Watson statistic presented in the **Figure 5** shows that no correlation can be observed between the experimental and calculated values so there is no evidence of correlation in the residuals' series, and therefore there is no accumulation of experimental error [**19**].

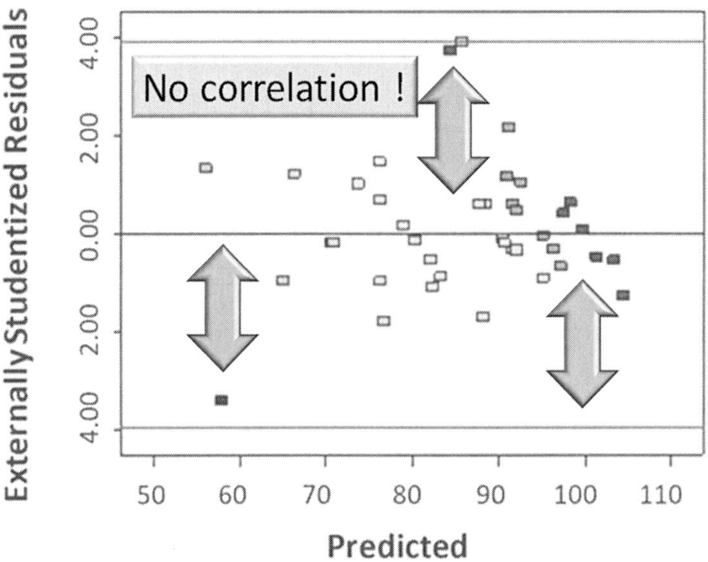

Figure 3.5. Residual correlation: q(experimental)–q(calculated).

Figure 3.6 offers a visual representation of the distinctive interactions among parameters that exert an influence on the system outcomes.

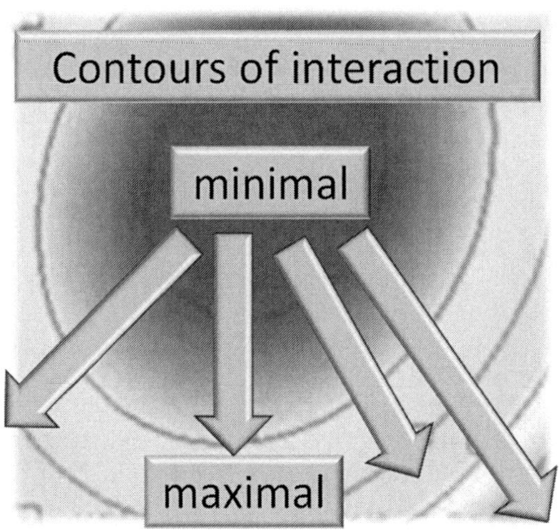

Figure 3.6. Effects of process parameters on water vapor permeability

The model obtained by optimization is shown in **Figure 3.7**,

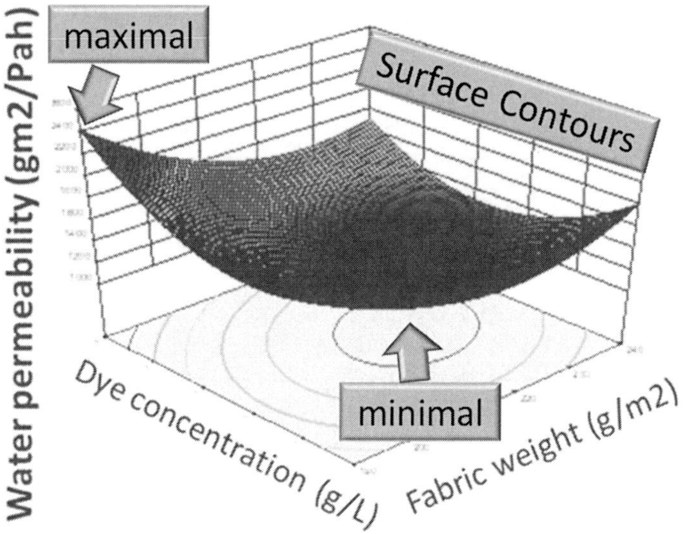

Figure 3.7. Effect of fabric weight and the dye concentration on water vapor permeability.

Notably, the input parameters, serve as independent variables of potential significance. It is crucial to recognize that the interactions among specific combinations of these process parameters can further impact the resultant output outcomes.

This graphical overview provides valuable insights into the intricate relationships and interplays that contribute to shaping the system's behaviour and responses.

Response Surface Methodology

Resistance to water wetting was effectively achieved using both Sevophob HFK–F and Tubiquard SCS–F, as they effectively reduced the surface energy of the fabric, preventing water from wetting the garment. While alternative finishers like waxes, oils, and silicones could produce similar effects, they may not possess the same level of repellence against substances like oil, sand, or lotion compounds.

Fluorocarbon compounds like Sevophob HFK–F and Tubiquard SCS–F were chosen due to their remarkable ability to repel both oil and water, a crucial attribute for military garment finishing. However, the eight-carbon atom composition of Sevophob HFK-F raised environmental concerns, necessitating the development of an equally efficient process using the six-carbon atom Tubiquard SCS–F.

Zahid et al. highlighted the frequent contact of textile materials with human skin and stressed the importance of non-toxic, biocompatible treatments that adhere to stringent health standards. Given the substantial amounts of water, chemicals, and reagents used in the textile industry, scalable, sustainable, and eco-friendly treatments are imperative. Consequently, eco-friendly processes are gaining traction and adoption.

Furthermore, Zahid et al.'s review article emphasized that while C8 fluorinated polymers are highly effective in rendering textiles water or oil repellent, their health and environmental risks have led to bans. As a result, C8-free alternatives for non-wettable treatments present promising commercialization prospects. The review also outlined future strategies and novel materials that hold the potential to transform non-wettable textile processes into entirely sustainable technologies.

In this work, the model was used to find the manner in which the parameters need to be varied in order to achieve the optimal solution for obtaining hydrophobic properties with less harmful reagents that contain six C atoms.

The quadratic model is shown in **Figure 3.8**.

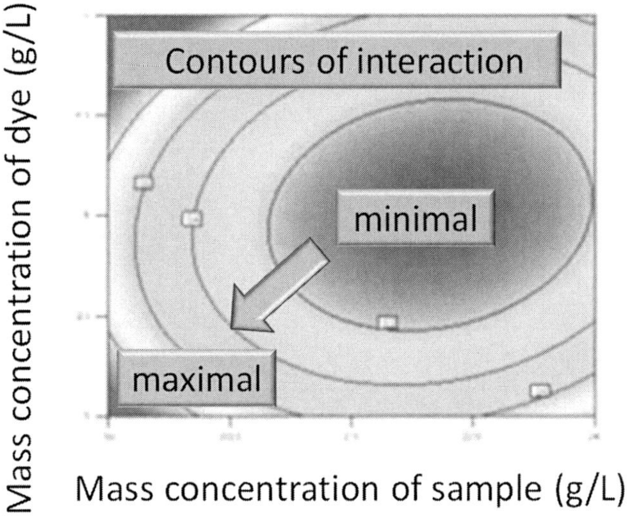

Figure 3.8. Surface contour plots for resistance to water wetting at optimal values

The surface contour plots illustrate the interactions between different industrial process variables, forming elliptical patterns. The central point represents the point where the contour's slope is zero in all directions.

The surface confined within the smallest curve of the contour diagram indicates the minimal predicted response yield. Therefore, the optimal and maximized solutions are located outside this area, as depicted in Figure 3.8.

The analysis of the results presented in Figure 3.8 highlights the substantial influence of process parameters on the outcomes. The figure demonstrates that increasing the concentration of hydrophobic compounds, dye concentration, and pressure contributes to the enhancement of water vapor permeability. Conversely, reducing the garment weight improves its efficiency. Furthermore, elevating the temperature enhances water vapor permeability but reduces resistance to water wetting. These findings can be explained by the fact that optimal coating finishing occurs under high reagent concentrations and stringent process conditions.

The statistical analysis of this model led to the identification of the optimal solution for maximizing water vapor permeability. Subsequently, additional experiments were conducted under these optimized conditions. The outcomes predicted by the Design of Experiment (DoE) were then compared to the experimental results, as depicted in Table 3.3. This table presents the results of verification experiments conducted at the optimal solutions for three different types of textile fabrics, each with a weight of 190 g/m^2.

Table 3.3. Verification of experiments and design constrains

Model checking by comparison of predicted and experimental data							
A	B	C	D	E	F	Predicted	Experiment
190	16.9	41.1	169	1.05	S	2670	2609

Constraints						
Name	Goal	Lower Limit	Upper Limit	Lower Weight	Upper Weight	Importance
A: fabric weight	range	190	240	1	1	3
B: dye concentration	range	10	60	1	1	3
C: hydrophobic concentration	range	35	70	1	1	3
D:Temperature	range	150	170	1	1	3
E: pressure	range	1	2	1	1	3

F: type of the hydrophobic compound	range	S	T	1	1	3
WVP	Max.	1196	6720	1	1	3

The table reveals that two optimal solutions were achieved using eight C atoms, while the other two were achieved with six C atoms. Notably, this outcome surpassed all preliminary tests for both six C atoms and eight C atoms by a remarkable 21.15%. Moreover, comparing the optimal result of 2620 g/m2 with the statistical mean value obtained solely for six C atoms (1726.86 g/m2), the global optimum demonstrated a significant improvement of 51.72%. This emphasizes that the industrial process can be executed under the presented variable parameters, yielding satisfying results that are both ecologically and economically viable.

The excellent resistance to water wetting endured even after undergoing five washing cycles, representing an outstanding accomplishment. Without the optimization, the resistance to water wetting effects would diminish to 50–70%, whereas our optimized process-maintained resistance to water wetting at a high level (90–100%). Figure 3.9 depicts the desirability for each factor and all responses individually for the selected optimal solution. Further underscoring the accuracy of our findings, Table 3 indicates an error of ±1.96% for resistance to water wetting and an error of ±2.28% for water vapor permeability, both with a 95% confidence level (i.e., 94 ± 0.52%).

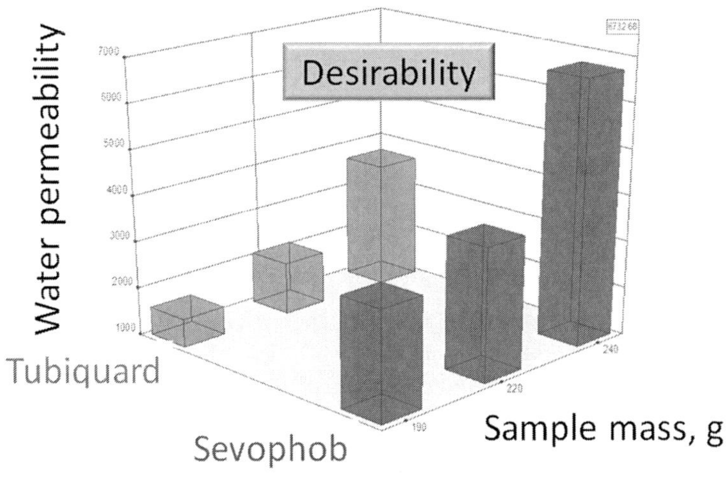

Figure 3.9. Desirability for each factor and each response individually

The verified optimized solution of the model responses of water vapor permeability and resistance to water wetting is shown in **Figure 3.10**.

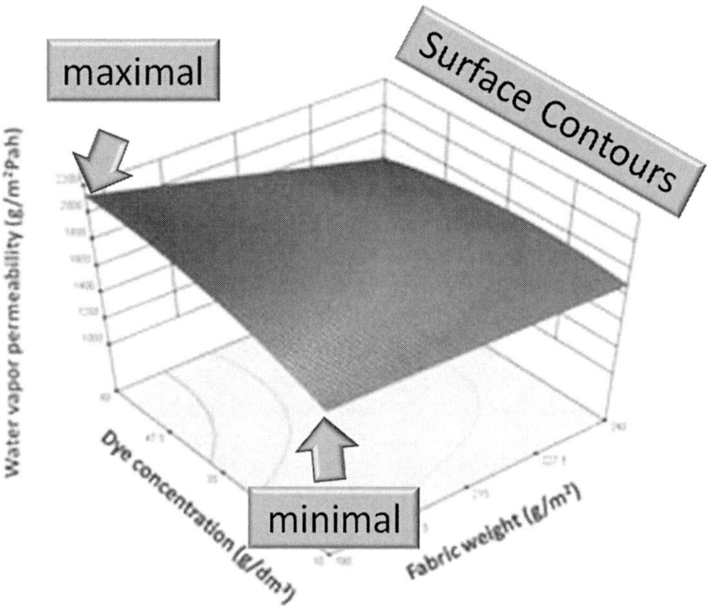

Figure 3.10. Response surface of the Central composite design

Utilizing the optimization model depicted in Figure 10, the predicted and verified optima for the responses (water vapor permeability and resistance to water wetting) were compared by assessing the concurrence between the predicted outcomes and the new experimental results.

An ecologically favourable optimal process involving a six C atoms fluorocarbon (Tubiquard, 68.802 g/L) outperformed all test outcomes by a substantial 21.15%. This achievement was realized at specific conditions: 154.3 °C, 1.05 bar pressure, 56.07 g/L dye concentration, and 220 g/m2 fabric weight. Remarkably, this optimal solution surpassed the statistical mean for six C atoms by an impressive 51.72%.

Additionally, an optimal solution employing an eight C atoms hydrophobic compound resulted in a water vapor permeability of 2609 g/m2. This achievement was attained under conditions of 152.5 °C temperature, 1.9 bar pressure, 38.815 g/L Sevophob HFK-F concentration, 11.1 g/L dye concentration on 240 g/m2 fabric weight.

Notably, this optimal solution exceeded the statistical mean of all test results involving eight C atoms (1619.2 g/m2) by an outstanding 61.12%.

From these findings, it can be deduced that Design of Experiment is an exceptional tool for optimizing complex multi-parameter systems. By conducting a fraction of the experiments required to estimate main effects and parameter interactions efficiently, it offers a highly effective approach, particularly in scenarios with a high number of factors [27].

> The presented work shows that Design of Experiment is a convivial tool for optimizing the modification of a surface since the influence of the various process parameters can be easily investigated. In this work, fabric weight, dye concentration, hydrophobic reagent concentration, temperature, pressure, and the type of the hydrophobic compound, have been investigated to determine the optimal conditions.

The validity of the regression equation has been rigorously assessed through a statistical approach, leading to the following noteworthy conclusions: *Sevophob HFK–F* and *Tubiquard SCS–F* emerge as effective hydrophobic reagents, with *Sevophob HFK–F* exhibiting superior efficiency. However, the ecological implications render *Sevophob HFK–F* unacceptable for use.

A Central Composite Design of Experiments was skilfully employed, involving 42 preliminary experiments. This approach enabled the investigation of six critical process parameters within a laboratory-scale optimization framework. The aim was to explore an alternative solution using *Tubiquard* SCS-F with six C atoms, addressing the ecological concerns. An ecologically favourable optimal solution was achieved employing a six C atoms fluorocarbon (*Tubiquard*) at a concentration of 68.802 g/L. This innovative approach surpassed all test results by an impressive margin of 21.15%. The optimal conditions were found at 154.3 °C temperature, 1.05 bar pressure, 56.07 g/L dye concentration, and a fabric weight of 220 g/m^2.

In light of these findings, it is evident that efficient water repellence can be successfully achieved using six C fluorocarbons. Moreover, the substitution of ecologically harmful and prohibited hydrophobic compounds containing eight C atoms can be effectively accomplished by employing industry-acceptable reagents. This research underscores the feasibility of achieving both performance and ecological compatibility within the realm of hydrophobic finishing processes.

The anticipated outcomes of this exploration are poised to unveil compelling insights into the influence of process parameters. Specifically, it is expected that increased pressure, elevated concentration of hydrophobic compounds, and higher dye concentrations will collectively enhance water vapor permeability. Conversely, a reduction in weight will likely amplify efficiency. Intriguingly, temperature escalation is anticipated to bolster water vapor permeability, albeit at the cost of diminished resistance to water wetting.

References

1. Sayed, U.; Dabhi, P. Finishing of textiles with fluorocarbons. In *The Textile Institute Book Series Waterproof and Water Repellent Textiles and Clothing, Chapter 6*; Williams, J., Ed.; Mahendra Publications; Woodhead Publishing: Cambridge, UK; Sawston, UK, 2014; pp. 139–153. [**Google Scholar**]
2. Rezić, I.; Krstić, D.; Bokić, L. Ultrasonic extraction of resins from an historical textile. *Ultrason. Sonochem.* **2008**, *15*, 21–24. [**Google Scholar**] [**CrossRef**] [**PubMed**]
3. Audenaert, F.; Lens, H.; Rolly, D.; Vander Elst, P. Fluoro-chemical textile repellents—Synthesis, and applications: A 3M perspective. *J. Text. Inst.* **1999**, *90*, 76–94. [**Google Scholar**] [**CrossRef**]
4. Schindler, W.; Hauser, P. *Chemical Finishing of Textiles*; Woodhead Publishing Ltd.: Boca Raton, FL, USA; Cambridge, UK, 2004; pp. 74–91. [**Google Scholar**]
5. Kissa, E.; Lewin, M.; Sello, S. *Handbook of Fiber Science and Technology, Chemical Processing of Fibers and Fabrics, Part B Functional Finishes*; Marcel Dekker: New York, NY, USA, 1984; Volume 2, p. 143. [**Google Scholar**]
6. Holmes, D.; Horrocks, A.; Anand, S. (Eds.) *Handbook of Technical Textiles*; Woodhead Publishing Ltd.: Cambridge, UK, 2000; p. 461. [**Google Scholar**]
7. Lu, D.; Sha, S.; Luo, J.; Huang, Z.; Zhang Jackie, X. Treatment train approaches for the remediation of per- and polyfluoroalkyl substances PFAS: A. critical review. *J. Hazard. Mater.* **2020**, *386*, 121963. [**Google Scholar**] [**CrossRef**] [**PubMed**]
8. Gibson, P. Water-repellent Treatment on Military Uniform Fabrics: Physiological and Comfort. *J. Ind. Text.* **2008**, *38*, 43–54. [**Google Scholar**] [**CrossRef**]
9. Murray, C.C.; Vatankhah, H.; McDonough, C.A.; Nickerson, A.; Hedtke, T.T.; Higgins, C.P.; Bellona, C.L. Removal of per- and polyfluoroalkyl substances using super-fine powder activated carbon and ceramic membrane filtration. *J. Hazard. Mater.* **2019**, *366*, 160–168. [**Google Scholar**] [**CrossRef**]

10. Zahid, M.; Heredia-Guerrero, J.A.; Athanassiou, A.; Bayer, I.S. Robust water repellent treatment for woven cotton fabrics with eco-friendly polymers. *Chem. Eng. J.* **2017**, *319*, 321–332. [**Google Scholar**] [**CrossRef**]
11. Moussa, A.; Marzoug, I.B.; Bouchereb, H. Development and optimisation of waterproof breathable double-sided knitting using a factorial experimental design. *J. Ind. Text.* **2015**, *45*, 437–466. [**Google Scholar**] [**CrossRef**]
12. Ravindra, D.; Kale, D.; Vade, A.; Potdar, T. Optimization study for Waterproof breathable Polyester fabric. *Int. J. Innov. Res. Technol.* **2016**, *3*, 16–24. [**Google Scholar**]
13. Huo, L.; Huang, X.; Li, J.; Guo, Z.; Gao, Q.; Hu, M.; Xue, H.; Gao, J. Superhydrophobic and multi-responsive fabric composite with excellent electro-photo-thermal effect and electromagnetic interference shielding performance. *Chem. Eng. J.* **2019**, 123537, in press, corrected proof. [**Google Scholar**] [**CrossRef**]
14. Peng, W.; Qin, H.; Zhao, M.; Zhao, X.; Guo, Z. Creation of a multifunctional superhydrophobic coating for composite insulators. *Chem. Eng. J.* **2018**, *352*, 774–781. [**Google Scholar**] [**CrossRef**]
15. Wang, J.; He, J.; Ma, L.; Zhang, Y.; Shen, L.; Xiong, S.; Li, K.; Qu, M. Multifunctional conductive cellulose fabric with flexibility, superamphiphobicity and flame-retardancy for all-weather wearable smart electronic textiles and high-temperature warning device. *Chem. Eng. J.* **2020**, *390*, 124508. [**Google Scholar**] [**CrossRef**]
16. Nabil, B.; Christine, C.; Julien, V.; Abdelkrim, A. Polyfunctional cotton fabrics with catalytic activity and antibacterial capacity. *Chem. Eng. J.* **2018**, *351*, 328–339. [**Google Scholar**] [**CrossRef**]
17. Rezić, I. Determination of engineered nanoparticles on textiles and in textile wastewaters. *TrAC Trends Anal. Chem.* **2011**, *30*, 1159–1167. [**Google Scholar**] [**CrossRef**]
18. Mukhopadhyay, A.; Midha, V.K. A Review on Designing the Waterproof Breathable Fabrics Part I: Fundamental Principles and Designing Aspects of Breathable Fabrics. *J. Ind. Text.* **2008**, *37*, 225–262. [**Google Scholar**] [**CrossRef**]
19. Coronado, M.; Segadães, A.M.; Andrés, A. Using mixture design of experiments to assess the environmental impact of clay-based structural ceramics containing foundry wastes. *J. Hazard. Mater.* **2015**, *299*, 529–539. [**Google Scholar**] [**CrossRef**] [**PubMed**]
20. Wahla, A.Q.; Iqbal, S.; Anwar, S.; Firdous, S.; Mueller, J.A. Optimizing the metribuzin degrading potential of a novel bacterial consortium based on Taguchi design of experiment. *J. Hazard. Mater.* **2019**, *366*, 1–9. [**Google Scholar**] [**CrossRef**]

21. Rezić, I. Prediction of the surface tension of surfactants mixtures for detergent formulation using Design Expert software. *Mon. Chem.* **2011**, *142*, 1219–1225. [**Google Scholar**] [**CrossRef**]
22. Rezić, T.; Rezić, I.; Blaženović, I.; Šantek, B. Optimization of corrosion process of stainless-steel coating during cleaning in steel brewery tanks. *Mater. Corros.* **2013**, *64*, 321–327. [**Google Scholar**] [**CrossRef**]
23. Andlar, M.; Rezić, I.; Oros, D.; Kracher, D.; Ludwig, R.; Rezić, T.; Šantek, B. Optimization of enzymatic sugar beet hydrolysis in a horizontal rotating tubular bioreactor. *J. Chem. Technol. Biotechnol.* **2017**, *92*, 623–632. [**Google Scholar**] [**CrossRef**]
24. United States Environmental Protection Agency. *EPA's Per- and Polyfluoroalkyl Substances PFAS Action Plan*; EPA 823R18004; United States Environmental Protection Agency: Washington, DC, USA, 2019. Available online: **https://www.epa.gov/pfas** (accessed on 2 May 2020).
25. Arabuli, S.; Vlasenko, V.; Havelka, A.; Kus, Z. Analysis of Modern Methods for Measuring Vapor Permeability Properties of Textiles. In Proceedings of the 7th International Conference—TEXSCI, Liberec, Czech Republic, 6–8 September 2010. [**Google Scholar**]
26. *ISO 4920:2012 Textile Fabrics—Determination of Resistance to Surface Wetting Spray Test*; International Organization for Standardization: Geneva, Switzerland, 2012.
27. Rezić, I. Optimization of ultrasonic extraction of 23 elements from cotton. *Ultrason. Sonochem.* **2009**, *16*, 63–69. [**Google Scholar**] [**CrossRef**]
28. Zahid, M.; Mazzon, G.; Athanassiou, A.; Bayer, I.S. Environmentally benign non-wettable textile treatments: A review of recent state-of-the-art. *Adv. Colloid Interface Sci.* **2019**, *270*, 216–250. [**Google Scholar**] [**CrossRef**] [**PubMed**]

CHAPTER FOUR

ANTIMICROBIAL COATINGS[1]

Introduction

The current landscape of antimicrobial research has placed a strong focus on investigating the *in vitro* antimicrobial activity of colloidal nanoparticle solutions against a range of model organisms, encompassing both gram-positive and gram-negative bacteria, as well as fungal species. These studies have extended to include specific strains of Staphylococcus aureus, encompassing both methicillin-sensitive (MSSA) and methicillin-resistant (MRSA) variants. This chapter seeks to elucidate the findings of an antimicrobial investigation involving various metal and metal-oxide nanoparticles. These nanoparticles, including Ag 10 nm, Ag 40 nm, Al2O3 100 nm, Pt 4 nm, TiO2 100 nm, Y2O3 100 nm, ZnO 100 nm, and ZrO2 100 nm, are potential candidates for utilization as coatings on biodegradable polymers produced through 3D printing. Specifically, applications such as catheters, disposable medical items, hospital bedding, antimicrobial linings, and bandages for chronic wounds are envisioned.

The evaluation of nanoparticle antimicrobial efficacy was undertaken through agar well diffusion assay and serial microdilution broth assay techniques. Additionally, a chromatographic analysis was conducted to detect trace amounts of elements, serving as a means to trace the presence of nanoparticles. Moreover, the feasibility of preparing the surface of biodegradable polymers for coating with antimicrobial nanoparticles was explored through the implementation of 3D printing via fused deposition methodology.

The in vitro findings emphasize the potent antimicrobial effects of specific nanoparticles against both MSSA and MRSA strains. Moreover, the nanoparticles demonstrated adaptability for application on diverse

---

[1] I. Rezić, M. Majdak, V. Ljoljić Bilić, I. Pokrovac, L. Martinaga, M. Somogyi Škoc, I. Kosalec, Development of Antibacterial Protective Coatings Active Against MSSA and MRSA on Biodegradable Polymers, Polymers 13 (2021) 659, 1-17 https://doi.org/10.3390/polym- 13040659

biopolymers. This research holds promise in advancing the development of effective antimicrobial coatings for a range of medical applications, contributing to the ongoing efforts in combating microbial infections and improving patient care. Projections suggest a concerning trend over the next three decades, where the threat posed by infections caused by antibiotic-resistant bacteria could potentially surpass the toll of cancer-related fatalities [1]. Despite advancements and a decline in infection rates since 2005, Staphylococcus aureus infections continue to impose significant morbidity and mortality burdens within the United States [2].

The integration of antimicrobial capabilities within biodegradable polymers, achieved through the incorporation of metal and metal oxide nanoparticles within their surface layer, holds immense potential in the realm of medicine and medical materials. These advanced materials offer a targeted approach to combatting methicillin-resistant Staphylococcus aureus (MRSA), particularly within industrial contexts. Notably, polymer materials that do not undergo traditional fibre production and spinning techniques, but are rather generated through alternative processes like additive technology or 3D printing, can be easily imbued with metal nanoparticles to confer antimicrobial properties. Such innovative materials find application in diverse medical scenarios, including catheters, disposable medical items, wound dressings, and dressings for chronic wounds. Moreover, these materials can be further adapted for use in the fabrication of protective masks and suits, extending their potential scope even further [3]. This multifaceted approach to integrating antimicrobial properties into polymer materials bears the promise of significantly enhancing infection control and prevention strategies, contributing to improved healthcare outcomes and public health.

Fight against super bacteria

This chapter delves into the subject of MRSA, a prominent member of the "super-bugs" category. This microorganism has garnered notoriety for its resistance to a broad spectrum of antibiotic-based penicillin drugs, such as methicillin, dicloxacillin, nafcillin, and oxacillin.

Belonging to the *Staphylococcus* family, MRSA is a Gram-positive bacterium characterized by its spherical morphology. Today, it stands as one of the most formidable pathogens globally, with a particularly concerning aspect being its associated fatality rate, which ranges from ten to thirty percent [4].

At the heart of this investigation lies the extraordinary antimicrobial potential of nanoparticles, a trait largely attributed to their nano-scale dimensions, typically ranging from one to one hundred nanometres. This size comparison vis-à-vis microorganisms highlights the nanoparticles' diminutiveness, rendering them substantially smaller than various microorganisms, including both Gram-positive and Gram-negative bacteria, as well as fungi. Consequently, the interaction mechanisms between nanoparticles and microorganisms have become a subject of intense research interest.

The intricate relationship between metal and metal oxide nanoparticles and microorganisms' manifests in two primary ways: interaction at the surface level and penetration through the microorganisms' cellular structures. Although the specific mechanisms governing the interaction between metal oxide nanoparticles and MRSA strains are still being explored, an array of nanoparticles has exhibited antimicrobial activity not only against MRSA but also against a diverse spectrum of other microorganisms, spanning bacteria and fungi alike [4]. This emerging understanding of nanoparticle-microorganism interactions underscores the potential for novel strategies in combating infectious diseases and inspires further investigation into harnessing these interactions for medical and industrial applications.

It is crucial to highlight that nanoparticles composed of metals and metal oxides can exhibit varying levels of toxicity to human cells. Notably, studies by Padmavathy and Vijayaraghavan have demonstrated the lack of biocompatibility between nanoparticles and human cells, making them suitable additives for polymers, textiles, and surfaces that come into direct contact with the human body [5]. Ongoing investigations in this domain are shedding further light on these interactions [6-17], underscoring their potential significance.

The integration of biodegradable polymers offers a sustainable avenue for producing disposable and environmentally friendly materials devoid of harm to the ecosystem and its inhabitants [18]. The use of products derived from biodegradable polymers is on the rise, growing by approximately 10 to 20% annually.

Among these materials, polylactide (PLA) stands out as one of the most prevalent. PLA, derived from natural sources like corn and potatoes, consists of lactic acid monomers and is synthesized through a two-step process involving polycondensation of lactic acid and the opening of the lactide ring. While PLA, like other aliphatic polyesters, including poly ε-caprolactone and polyhydroxy butyrate, exhibits biodegradability in both the human body and nature, its relatively high crystallinity and molecular weight contribute to a slower rate of biodegradation.

The medical applications of PLA date back to the 1980s, primarily involving its utilization as a carrier for efficient drug delivery within the body. PLA and its copolymers have shown promise for this purpose. Additionally, PLA has emerged as a suitable alternative to metal implants, such as rods, screws, and scaffolds, used for bone fixation and tissue healing. Remarkably, due to its biodegradability, PLA implants do not necessitate surgical removal, unlike traditional metal counterparts. PLA's compatibility with the human body has led to its adoption in surgical sutures, skin grafts, and other medical interventions. The advent of additive technology, commonly known as 3D printing, has expedited the fabrication of intricately designed objects using CAD modeling or computer scanning. Post-printing processes, including finishing and functionalization with antimicrobial coatings, further enhance the versatility of PLA-based materials. These coatings can be easily applied through techniques like dip-coating [18].

As the realm of nanotechnology and biodegradable polymers continues to evolve, their synergy offers novel avenues for producing safe, effective, and environmentally conscious materials with diverse applications in medicine, textiles, and beyond.

Antimicrobial enhancements of polymer materials through the incorporation of nanoparticles can be further optimized through ultrasonic treatment, as demonstrated by Abramova et al. In their study, they coated textiles with titanium and zinc oxide nanoparticles to explore the feasibility of creating antibacterial coatings on textile materials [19]. The results indicated a remarkable reduction of investigated microorganisms, such as Escherichia coli, by more than 99.99%. Similarly, Akhavan and Montazer conducted a study involving the simultaneous loading of $TiO2$ nanoparticles onto cotton using sonochemistry. This innovative approach led to the production of self-cleaning materials with UV protection properties [20].

Sonochemistry, a process involving the use of ultrasonic waves, has a significant impact on the mechanical properties of nanocomposite films [21, 22].

It has been observed that sonochemical irradiation not only enhances the mechanical properties of nanocomposite films but also facilitates the synthesis of nanoparticles at lower temperatures and in a more efficient manner [23]. The resulting polymers from these processes possess effective antimicrobial protection against model microorganisms, specifically Gram-positive bacteria (S. aureus), Gram-negative bacteria (E. coli), and fungi (Candida albicans). The inhibition zones for all tested microorganisms ranged from 3.0 to 3.3 mm [23]. Further developments in this area have explored the use of thorn-like nanoparticles, which have shown promising results due to their size and shape influencing antibacterial efficacy [24, 25]. It is evident that the toxicity and antibacterial effects of nanomaterials depend on various input process variables that can be effectively controlled, such as the chemical and morphological composition of nanoparticles, as well as their size and shape. This understanding underscores the potential for tailoring nanomaterial properties to achieve specific antimicrobial outcomes in polymer-based applications.

> Nanomaterial toxicity and antibacterial effects depend on different input process variables which we can easily control, such are the chemical and morphological composition of nanoparticles, their size and their shape.

Regrettably, certain nanoparticle shapes have demonstrated toxicity towards organisms like daphnids and other living beings [26]. When comparing the toxic effects of nanoparticles based on their size, it becomes evident that those with smaller diameters, such as nanoparticles measuring twenty to thirty nm, tend to induce more potent toxic effects compared to larger nanoparticles. This phenomenon can be attributed to the higher likelihood of smaller nanoparticles entering the cells of the organisms being investigated [27]. Metal nanoparticles can be effectively incorporated onto cellulose materials through a dip-coating process, yielding flexible, uniform, and cohesive coatings [28–31]. To accurately characterize metal nanoparticles, analytical methods that offer precise and reliable analysis of trace amounts are required. Spectroscopy and chromatography are two such methodologies. Chromatography, in particular, allows for the simultaneous separation, identification, and quantification of analytes. It can be performed using columns or thin-layer setups. Thin-layer chromatography (TLC) is often recommended due to its speed and simplicity. By manipulating stationary and mobile phases, tailored methods can be developed for monitoring and assessing specific components. Alongside ion chromatography, thin-layer chromatography stands out as a valuable technique for evaluating metal content on thin layers [38, 39].

In order to evaluate the impact of colloidal metal and metal-oxide nanoparticles, a comprehensive investigation was conducted on nine distinct model colloid nanoparticle systems: Ag 40 nm (20 ppm), Ag 10 nm (20 ppm), Pt 4 nm (at concentrations of 250, 225, and 100 ppm), ZnO 100 nm (at concentrations of 10% and 21%), Au 20 nm (20 ppm), TiO2 100 nm (33%), Al2O3 100 nm (20%), Y2O3 100 nm (at concentrations of 5% and 10%), and ZrO2 100 nm (5%). This assessment involved both agars well diffusion and serial two-fold microdilution assays4. The overarching objective of this research endeavour was twofold: the development of antimicrobial biodegradable polymers and the establishment of a methodology for characterizing metal nanoparticles.

To achieve these aims, two primary steps were pursued. First, thin layer chromatography (TLC) was examined as a potential analytical tool for the analysis of 60 different elements, primarily focusing on metal ions (as detailed in Table 4.1). Second, the antimicrobial effects of up to seven diverse nanoparticles—both metal and metal oxides—were investigated, as depicted in Tables 4.2 and 4.3. The TLC technique was tailored for the analysis of metal ions, which could be extracted from functionalized polymers through interactions with metal and metal oxide nanoparticles. These nanoparticles are often employed in the antimicrobial coating of biodegradable polymer samples.

Table 4.1 catalogues sixty metals that underwent investigation as potential antimicrobial agents against microorganisms through thin layer chromatography. During preliminary experiments, thirty-one distinct stationary phases were assessed, each comprising thin layers constructed from alumina oxide, cellulose, polyamide, and silica gel. These stationary phases were subjected to various organic solvents and solvent mixtures as mobile phases. Specifically, acetonitrile and acetyl acetone were compared against butanol and triethylamine, as well as ethylenediaminetetraacetic acid (EDTA), to optimize the chromatographic conditions for this analysis.

Furthermore, to enhance the chromatographic separation and analysis, specific inorganic compounds like hydrochloric acid (HCl) and water were incorporated into selected mobile phases. This was done to create optimal solvent mixtures that would facilitate effective separation and identification of the target metal ions. In total, a comprehensive array of nineteen distinct solvent mixtures were generated and evaluated during the preliminary stages of experimentation.

Table 4.1. Metals for production of nanoparticles

	Element	Symbol		Element	Symbol
1	Silver	Ag	31	Magnesium	Mg
2	Aluminium	Al	32	Molybdenum	Mo
3	Arsenic	As	33	Sodium	Na
4	Gold	Au	34	Niobium	Nb
5	Boron	B	35	Neodymium	Nd
6	Barium	Ba	36	Nickel	Ni
7	Beryllium	Be	37	Osmium	Os

8	Bismuth	Bi	38	Phosphor	P
9	Brome	Br	39	Lead	Pb
10	Calcium	Ca	40	Palladium	Pd
11	Cadmium	Cd	41	Platinum	Pt
12	Cobalt	Co	42	Rubidium	Rb
13	Chrome	Cr	43	Rhenium	Re
14	Cesium	Cs	44	Rhodium	Rh
15	Copper	Cu	45	Ruthenium	Ru
16	Dysprosium	Dy	46	Sulfur	S
17	Europium	Eu	47	Antimony	Sb
18	Iron	Fe	48	Scandium	Sc
19	Gallium	Ga	49	Selenium	Se
20	Gadolinium	Gd	50	Silica	Si
21	Germanium	Ge	51	Tin	Sn
22	Hafnium	Hf	52	Strontium	Sr
23	Mercury	Hg	53	Tantalum	Ta
24	Holmium	Ho	54	Tellurium	Te
25	Indium	In	55	Thorium	Th
26	Iridium	Ir	56	Titanium	Ti
27	Potassium	K	57	Thallium	Tl
28	Lithium	Li	58	Uranium	U
29	Lutetium	Lu	59	Vanadium	V
30	Manganese	Mn	60	Tungsten	W

Ultimately, the chromatographic methodology was fine-tuned and optimized to achieve successful separation and identification of all 60 targeted metal ions. In this optimized approach, the stationary phase consisted of silica gel, while the mobile phase incorporated a combination of three different solvents: acetonitrile (ACN), hydrochloric acid (HCl), and water (H2O). The proportions of these solvents in the mobile phase were determined through rigorous optimization, resulting in a calculated volume ratio of 60.00% ACN, 19.17% HCl, and 20.83% water.

This optimized chromatographic system was then utilized for the subsequent analyses, and the outcomes of these efforts are illustrated in Figures 4.1 and 4.2, which showcase the collected results and the successful separation and identification of the targeted metal ions.

Novel strategy for super bacteria

The subsequent phase in the fabrication of antimicrobial polymers involved the utilization of 3D printing technology to create surfaces that could subsequently be endowed with antimicrobial coatings. These coated surfaces were envisioned to serve as disposable items with significant applications in the medical field. Contemporary and advanced methods for producing small-scale biodegradable materials are increasingly finding widespread utility in various aspects of daily life. Moreover, additive technology, particularly 3D printing, allows for the precision crafting of specialized shapes following meticulous modeling and preparation. These shapes can then be further functionalized with metal coatings and metal nanoparticles to confer antimicrobial properties. The intended applications for such materials encompass catheters, consumables, dressings, wound dressings, as well as the potential for use in manufacturing protective masks and suits – essential items in today's medical landscape.

A comprehensive description of the surface modification procedure via the sol-gel approach has been documented in our prior research [47]. This prior study elucidates the methodology employed for the modification of polymer surfaces using ZnO nanoparticles. The process involves dip-coating the surface with a precursor compound called 3-glycidyloxypropyltrimethoxysilane (GLYMO, Sigma Aldrich, Darmstadt, Germany, Europe), with the addition of HCl as a catalyst. The nanoparticles, present in a sol state, are allowed to undergo gelation at ambient temperature before being subjected to a 24-hour drying period at room temperature. Following this, the material is heated to 100 °C for a duration of 60 minutes to further consolidate the coating.

The modified products underwent characterization using a variety of instrumental techniques, encompassing thin layer chromatography (TLC), scanning electron microscopy coupled with an energy-dispersive X-ray (SEM-EDX) detector (Tescan Vega, Brno, Czech Republic), and Fourier-transform infrared attenuated total reflection spectroscopy (FTIR-ATR) conducted with a Perkin Elmer instrument (Waltham, Massachusetts, USA) [47]. In the present study, the focus will be on showcasing the outcomes of the surface modification carried out using silver nanoparticles.

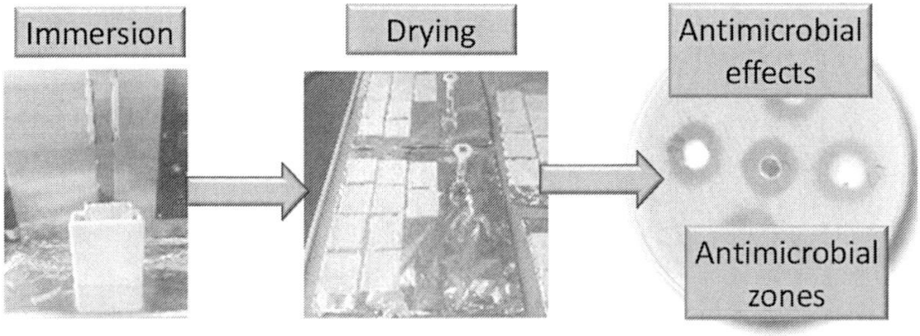

Figure 4.1. Immersion, drying and antimicrobial testing of samples during modification of surface

The samples that underwent coating were subjected to examination using a scanning electron microscope, specifically the "TESCAN VEGA TS5136LS" model equipped with an energy-dispersive X-ray spectroscopy (EDS) detector from Tescan Vega company located in Brno, Czech Republic. An SEM microphotograph of the modified antimicrobial cellulose material is presented in the Results section. For the purpose of spectroscopical and microscopical characterization, the following instrumentation was employed: a Fourier transform infrared spectrometer (Spectrum 100 FTIR) manufactured by Perkin Elmer in Waltham, Massachusetts, U.S.A. This instrument utilized KBr and Attenuated Total Reflectance (ATR) techniques to record spectra of cellulose materials in their solid state. The spectra of the samples were recorded over a frequency range spanning from 400 to 4000 cm−1 using the diffuse reflectance mode, with a resolution of 4 cm^{-1}.

The investigation into antimicrobial activity was conducted on a model microorganism, S. aureus, through a two-step process. The first step involved the agar well diffusion assay, followed by the serial microdilution broth assay. [32].

The evaluation of antimicrobial activity was carried out by measuring the diameters of zones of growth inhibition (Z.I.; d, mm), as shown in Table 4.2. In the second phase of the antimicrobial activity investigation, a serial microdilution broth assay was employed, following the procedures outlined in reference [33]. Notably, a significant modification was introduced, involving the replacement of Mueller–Hinton broth with physiological saline, as previously described [42]. This modification was implemented to mitigate any potential interference caused by nanosized colloidal metal and metal oxide particles with the diverse protein contents present in the original broth [42]. The investigation adhered to the standard protocol of serial two-fold micro-dilution, with incubation at 37 °C and a duration of 18-24 hours [33]. Standard reference materials of nanoparticles in colloidal form were included in the serial and two-fold dilution sequences.

The chromatographic investigation encompassed data collected from 31 different types of stationary phases, including cellulose, silica gel, polyamide, and alumina. Multiple mobile phases were tested, comprising various mixtures of inorganic and organic solvents, such as acetonitrile, acetyl acetone, butanol, triethylamine, and ethylenediaminetetraacetic acid. The optimized system for detecting metal ions involved silica gel as the stationary phase and a mobile phase composed of acetonitrile: hydrochloric acid: water, with a volume ratio of 60.00: 19.17: 20.83. The optimization of this system was achieved through 31 preliminary experiments. This optimized system was then applied to test all metals, and the results are detailed in the subsequent paragraph.

Figures 4.2 and 4.3 visually depict the distribution of metals separated and determined by the cellulose and silica gel stationary phases.

The examined elements exhibit potential antimicrobial properties when present in the form of metal or metal oxide nanoparticles and coated onto biodegradable polymers. The outcomes of chromatographic analyses featuring metal ions including silver, aluminum, arsenic, gold, bismuth, cadmium, cobalt, chromium, copper, iron, mercury, manganese, nickel, lead, antimony, silicon, tin, and zinc are illustrated in Figures 1 and 2. Throughout the experimentation, a developer mixture composed of ACN, HCl, and H2O in a ratio of 72:25:23 was employed. Notably, the most favorable separation outcomes were achieved with plates 1 (Polygram Cel 300), 8 (Silica gel), 26 (Cellulose F), as well as hydrophobic plates 19 (HPTLC RP-18 F254), 21 (HPTLC), 22 (HPTLC), and 23 (HPTLC RP18). Regarding the hydrophobic plates, it is noteworthy that they all exhibited similar results.

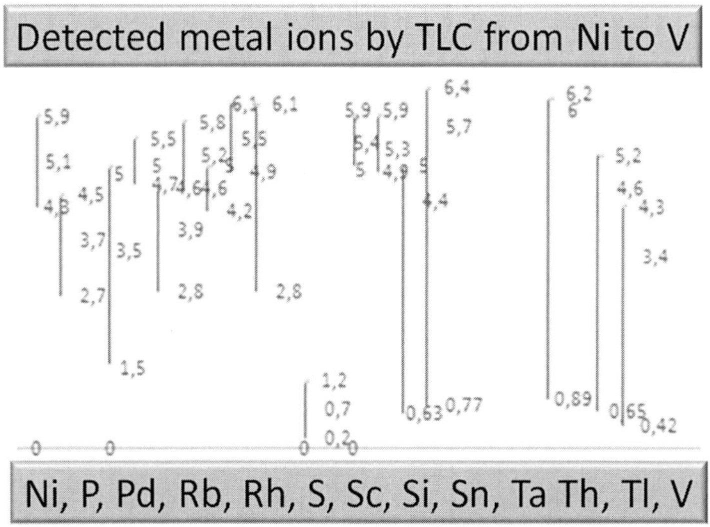

Figure 4.2. Metal ions detected by thin layer chromatography from Ni to V[4]

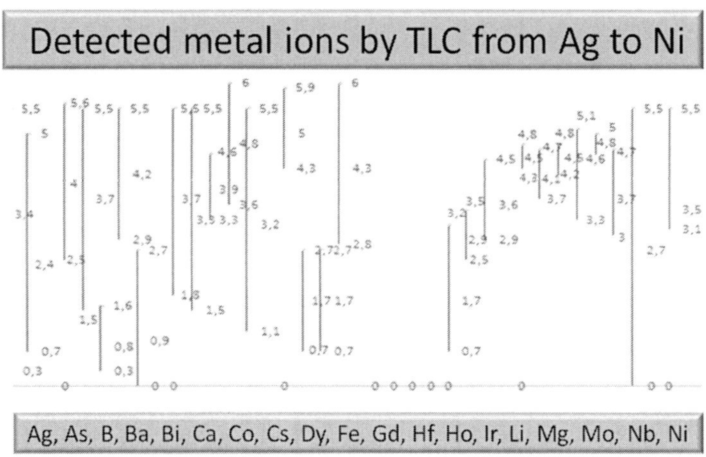

Figure 4.3. Metal ions detected by thin layer chromatography from Ag to Ni[4]

3D printed antibacterial items

The process of designing and preparing biodegradable polymer materials, such as polylactide, for 3D printing was executed in multiple sequential stages, outlined in Figures 4.4 to 4.7. These figures provide a comprehensive visual depiction of the progression involved in creating biodegradable polymer carriers intended for coating with antibacterial nanoparticles, as detailed in references [40-48]. It's worth noting that these materials can be adapted and manufactured in various configurations suitable for applications such as catheters, consumables, coatings, and bags.

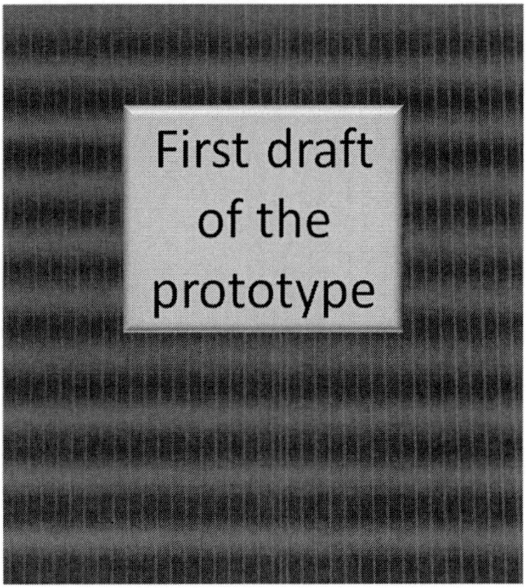

Figure 4.4: The first step of modeling by Blender computer programme

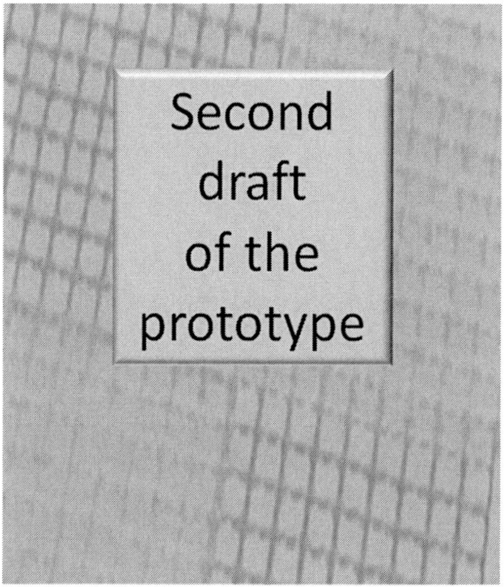

Figure 4.5: The second step of the modeling by Cura programme

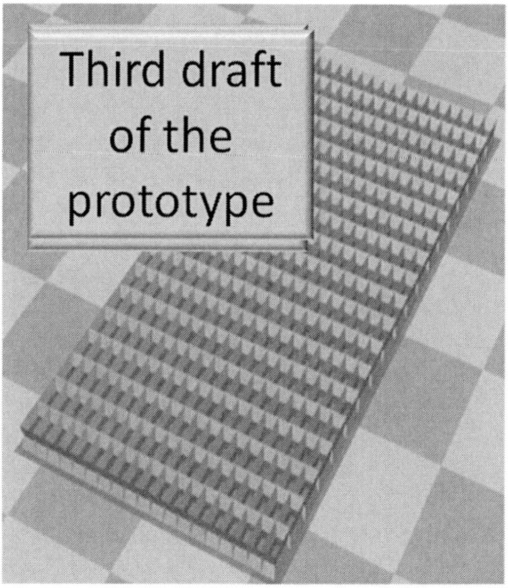

Figure 4.6: The third step of the modeling by Ultimaker

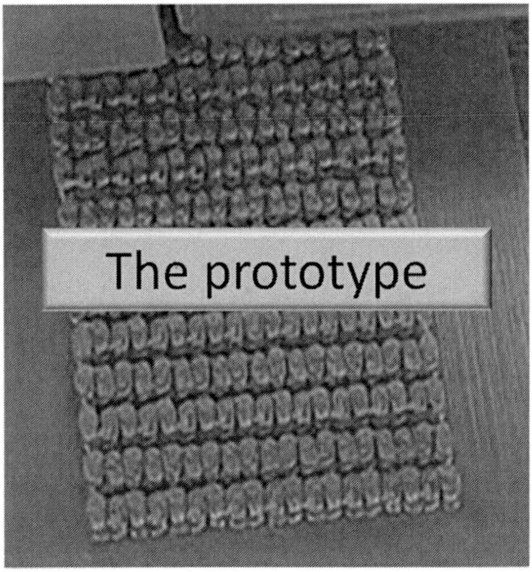

Figure 4.7: 3D printing of the prototype

The tiles produced through the 3D printing process, as depicted in images 4.3 to 4.6, exhibit a relatively modest resolution, a characteristic determined by the limitations of the printer itself. As a consequence, achieving an ultra-fine lattice structure with exceptionally high resolution is not attainable. These printed tiles exhibit an uneven surface, resulting in a rough texture, while the cross-sectional profile resembles that of a "sandwich". Despite these characteristics, these printed plates are primed for subsequent treatment through the sol-gel process, facilitating the functionalization of biodegradable polymers into antimicrobial materials.

For the purpose of spectroscopic characterization, Fourier-transform infrared spectrometry (Spectrum 100 FTIR, Perkin Elmer, Waltham, Massachusetts) is employed as a robust and reliable technique. This methodology proves effective in detecting the presence of distinct functional groups on the surface of the polymer, as demonstrated in Figure 8. The selection of this technique was based on its exceptional capability to identify differences in newly formed functional groups within the examined solid samples [47].

In this phase of the study, the focus was on examining biodegradable cellulose polymers that had been subjected to modification with silver nanoparticles. These samples were subsequently subjected to microscopic characterization using a scanning electron microscope with an energy-dispersive X-ray detector (SEM-EDX) at magnifications ranging from 80×

to 100× (as illustrated in Figure 4.9). It is important to note that all nanoparticles employed in this research were in the form of colloidally stable solutions or suspensions.

The nanoparticles were procured in certified forms, ensuring their chemical composition and concentrations were well-defined and validated. Detailed information regarding the certified chemical composition and concentrations of the nanoparticles can be found in Tables 4.2 to 4.4. This rigorous approach to nanoparticle acquisition and characterization contributes to the reliability and robustness of the study's findings.

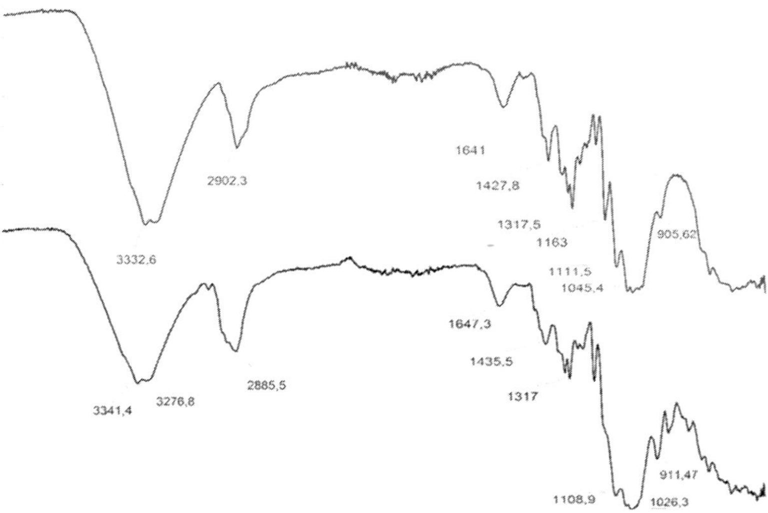

Figure 4.8. Fourier-transform infrared spectra until 1000 cm of sample

Figure 4.8 and the subsequent analyses involving peaks corresponding to epoxy groups, Si–O groups, and methoxy groups. The micro-photographical characterization through SEM-EDX and the interpretation are presented in Figure 4.9. The conclusion highlights the success of the dip-coating process in achieving a uniform and consistent coating of Ag nanoparticles. Overall, this chapter captures and highlights the important details and outcomes of the presented research.

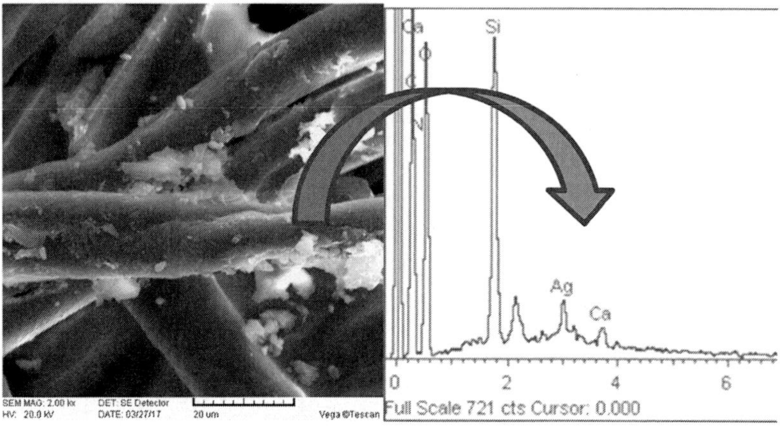

Figure 4.9. A) SEM microphotograph, **B**) SEM-EDX spectra of Ag coating[4].

The mechanism of MRSA antibiotic resistance does not seem to apply to nano-sized ZnO, as evidenced in the literature. However, our study[4], a difference in MIC and MBC values was observed in comparison to the MSSA strain, with higher values for MRSA, showing an MIC of 3.28 ± 0.55 ppm and an MBC of 3.28 ± 1.89 ppm [50]. Conversely, for TiO_2 (100 nm) nanoparticles, the MIC value for MSSA was twice as high as that for MRSA. A similar trend was observed when comparing the MBC values, which were consistently higher for MRSA strains than for MSSA strains. Specifically, the MBC values were 23.43 times higher for MRSA than MSSA when using ZnO (100 nm) nanoparticles, 8.07 times higher with Ag (10 nm) nanoparticles, and only 0.1 times higher with TiO_2 (100 nm) nanoparticles.

An effective antimicrobial strategy involves the application of antimicrobial colloidal nanoparticles. Li and colleagues investigated the antibacterial activity and mechanism of silver nanoparticles on *S. aureus* [44].

Their findings revealed a minimal bactericidal concentration (MBC) of 20 μg/mL. In comparison, Mirzajani and coauthors investigated silver nanoparticles against *S. aureus* strain PTCC1431 and found that nanoparticles at a concentration of 4 μg/mL completely inhibited bacterial growth [45]. Exposure of *S. aureus* to silver nanoparticles at a higher concentration (50 μg/mL) for 6 hours resulted in DNA damage, followed by cell wall rupture after 12 hours. This interaction led to the release of cellular contents into the surroundings, ultimately resulting in total cell collapse [44]. Grigoreva et al. further confirmed this direct interaction between silver nanoparticles and *S. aureus* strain's macromolecular structures [46]. The results of this study align with the literature, highlighting silver and ZnO nanoparticles as promising candidates for antibacterial medical materials produced from biodegradable polymers.

This interdisciplinary research has highlighted various aspects of developing optimal nanotechnological medical solutions for tackling bacterial infections. With the surge in demand for antimicrobial materials due to the COVID-19 pandemic and increased hospitalizations, this study sought to address crucial questions regarding the functionalization and preparation of antimicrobial coatings effective against *S. aureus* infections or colonization, including MSSA and MRSA strains. The study demonstrated the antimicrobial effects of numerous metal and metal oxide nanoparticles in vitro, and the potential of 3D printing to create customized polymer carriers for medical applications. In conclusion, colloidal nanoparticles such as silver (10 nm) and zinc oxide (100 nm) emerged as promising candidates for medical materials. Additionally, the study attempted to develop a chromatographic methodology for simultaneous separation and determination of trace analytes, representing an initial step with potential for further research.

References

1. World Health Organization. Antimicrobial Resistance Global Report on Surveillance 2014. Available online: https//www.who.int/drugresistance/documents/surveillancereport/en/(accessed on January 2020).
2. Van Kourtis; A.P. Hatfield K.; Baggs J.; Mu Y.; See I.; Epson E.; Nadle J.; Kainer M.A; Dumyati G.; Petit S.; Ray S.M.; Emerging Infections Program MRSA author group; D. Ham; C. Capers; H. Ewing; N. Coffin; L. C. McDonald; J.. Jernigan; D. Cardo, Vital Signs: Epidemiology and Recent Trends in Methicillin-Resistant and in Methicillin-Susceptible *Staphylococcus aureus* Bloodstream Infections — United States. *Morbid. Morta. Week. Rep.* **2019,** 68, 214–219.
3. Rahman Bhuiyan M.A., Wang L.; Shaid A., Shanks R.A.; Ding J., Advances and applications of chemical protective clothing system. *J. Ind. Text.* **2019**, 49, 97–138.
4. Delaney, J.C., Schneider-Lindner, V., Brassard, P. et al. Mortality after infection with methicillin-resistant *Staphylococcus aureus* (MRSA) diagnosed in the community. *BMC Med* **2008**, *6*, 2.

5. Padmavathy, N.; Vijayaraghavan, R. Enhanced bioactivity of ZnO nanoparticles-an antimicrobial study. *Sci. Technol. Adv. Mater.* **2008**, *9*, 035004.
6. Saraf, R. Cost effective and monodispersed zinc oxide nanoparticles synthesis. *Int. J. Adv. Appl. Sci.* **2013**, *2*, 85–88.
7. Liu, Q.; Zhang, M.; Fang Zx Rong, X.H. Effect of homogenization and ultrasonication on the physical properties of insoluble wheat bran fibres. *J. Sci. Food Agric.* **2014**, *94*, 2547–2554.
8. Beyth, N.; Houri-Haddad, Y.; Domb, A.; Khan, W.; Hazan, R. Alternative Antimicrobial Approach Nano-Antimicrobial Materials. *Complement. Altern. Med.* **2015**, *2015*, 246012.
9. Dizaj, S.M.; Lotpoura, F.; Barzegar-Jalali, M.; Zarrintana, M.H.; Adibkiab, K. Antimicrobial activity of the metals and metal oxide nanoparticles. *Mater. Sci. Eng. C* **2014**, *44*, 278–284.
10. Emami-Karvani, Z.; Chehrazi, P. Antibacterial activity of ZnO nanoparticle on Gram-positive and Gram- negative bacteria. *Afr. J. Microbiol. Res.* **2011**, *5*, 1368–1373.
11. Rasmussen, J.W.; Martinez, E.; Louka, P.; Wingett, D.G. Zinc oxide nanoparticles for selective destruction of tumor cells and potential for drug delivery applications. *Expert Opin. Drug Deliv.* **2010**, *7*, 1063–1077.
12. Brayner, R.; Ferrari-Iliou, R.; Brivois, N.; Djediat, S.; Benedetti, M.F.; Fievet, F. Toxicological impact studies based on *Escherichia coli* bacteria in ultrafine ZnO nanoparticles colloidal medium. *Nano Lett.* **2006**, *6*, 866–870.
13. Jones, N.; Ray, B.; Ranjit, K.T.; Manna, A.C. Antibacterial activity of ZnO nanoparticle suspensions on a broad spectrum of microorganisms. *FEMS Microbiol. Lett.* **2008**, *279*, 71–76.
14. Jalal, R.; Goharshadi, E.K.; Abareshi, M.; Moosavi, M.; Yousefi, A.; Nancarrow, P. ZnO nanofluids: Green synthesis, characterization. *Mater. Chem. Phys.* **2008**, *121*, 198–201.
15. Raghupathi, K.R.; Koodali, R.T.; Manna, A.C. Size-dependent bacterial growth inhibition and mechanism of antibacterial activity of zinc oxide nanoparticles. *Langmuir* **2011**, *27*, 4020–4028.
16. Xie, Y.; He, Y.; Irwin, P.L.; Jin, T.; Shi, X. Combined Fluxomics and Transcriptomics Analysis of Glucose Catabolism via a Partially Cyclic Pentose Phosphate Pathway in *Gluconobacter oxydans* 621H. *Appl. Environ. Microbiol.* **2011**, *77*, 2325–2331.
17. Fan, Z.; Lu, J.G. Zinc oxide nanostructures: Synthesis and properties. *J. Nanosci. Nanotechnol.* **2005**, *5*, 1561–1573.

18. Y. Zhong, P. Godwin, Y. Jin, H.Xiao; Biodegradable polymers and green-based antimicrobial packaging materials: A mini-review. *Adv. Ind. Eng. Polym. Res*. 2020, 3, 27-35.
19. Abramova, A.V.; Abramova, V.O.; Bayazitova, V.M.; Voitova, Y.; Straumal, E.A.; Lermontov, S.A.; Cherdyntseva, T.A.; Braeutigam, P.; Weiße, M.; Günther, K. A sol-gel method for applying nanosized antibacterial particles to the surface of textile materials in an ultrasonic field. *Ultrason. Sonochem.* **2020**, *60*, 104788.
20. Akhavan, F.; Majid Montazer, S. In situ sonosynthesis of nano TiO_2 on cotton fabric. *Ultrason. Sonochem.* **2014**, *21*, 681–691.
21. Behzadnia, A.; Montazer, M.; MahmoudiRad, M. *In situ* photo sonosynthesis and characterize nonmetal/metal dual doped honeycomb-like ZnO nanocomposites on wool fabric. *Ultrason. Sonochem.* **2015**, *27*, 200–209.
22. Ahmadizadegan, H.; Esmaielzadeha, S.; Ranjbara, M.; Marzban, Z.; Ghavas, F. Synthesis and characterization of polyester bionanocomposite membrane with ultrasonic irradiation process for gas permeation and antibacterial activity. *Ultrason. Sonochem.* **2018**, *41*, 538–550.
23. Ghayempour, S.; Montazer, M. Ultrasound irradiation based *in-situ* synthesis of star-like *Tragacanth gum*/zinc oxide nanoparticles on cotton fabric. *Ultrason. Sonochem.* **2017**, *34*, 458–465.
24. Khan, M.F.; Ansari, A.H.; Hameedullah, M.; Ahmad, E.; Husain, F.M.; Zia, Q.; Baig, U.; Zaheer, M.R.; Alam, M.M.; Khan, A.M.; et al. Sol-gel synthesis of thorn-like ZnO nanoparticles endorsing mechanical stirring effect and their antimicrobial activities: Potential role as nano-antibiotics. *Nat. Sci. Rep.* **2016**, *6*, 27689, doi10.1038/srep27689.
25. Barata, C.; Varo, I.; Navarro, J.C.; Arun, S.; Porte, C. Antioxidant enzyme activities and lipid peroxidation in the freshwater cladoceran *Daphnia magna* exposed to redox cycling compounds. *Toxicol. Pharmacol.* **2005**, *140*, 175–186.
26. Liu, J.; Fan, D.; Wang, L.; Shi, L.; Ding, J.; Chen, Y.; Shen, S. Effects of ZnO, CuO, Au, and TiO_2 nanoparticles on *Daphnia magna* and early life stages of zebrafish *Danio rerio. Env. Protect. Eng.* **2014**, *40*, 139–1491.
27. Seabra, A.B.; Durán, N. Nanotoxicology of Metal Oxide Nanoparticles. *Metals* **2015**, *5*, 934–975.
28. Wang, N.; Magdassi, S.; Madnler, D.; Long, Y. Simple sol-gel process and one-step annealing of vanadium dioxide thin films: Synthesis and thermochromic properties. *Thin Solid Film.* **2013**, *534*, 594–598.

29. Yadav, A.; Prasad, V.; Kathe, A.A.; Raj, S.; Yadav, D.; Sundaramoorthy, C.; Vigneshwaran, N. Functional finishing in cotton fabrics using zinc oxide nanoparticles. *Bull. Mater. Sci.* **2006**, *29*, 641–645.
30. Vigneshwaran, N.; Kumar, S.; Kathe, A.A.; Varadarajan, P.V.; Prasad, V. Functional finishing of cotton fabrics using zinc oxide soluble starch nanocomposites. *Nanotechnology* **2006**, *17*, 5087–5095.
31. Rezić, I. Cellulosic fibers-biosorptive materials and indicators of heavy metals pollution. *Microchem. J.* **2013**, *107*, 63–69.
32. Council of Europe.; *European Pharmacopoeia* Commission, *European Pharmacopoeia*, 5th Edition.Council of Europe: Strasbourg, France, **2005**; 188–191.
33. European Committee for Antimicrobial Susceptibility Testing (EUCAST) of the European Society for Clinical Microbiology and Infectious Diseases (ESCMID). EUCAST Discussion Document E.Def.5.1. *Clin. Microbiol. Infec.* **2003**, *9*, 1–7.
34. Peran, J.; Ercegović Ražić, S.; Kosalec, I.; Ziberi, F. Antimicrobial Effectiveness of Cellulose based Fabrics treated with Silver Nitrate Solution using Plasma Processes.*Tekstilec* **2017**, *60*, 247–253.
35. Rezić, I. Optimization of ultrasonic extraction of 23 elements from cotton. *Ultrason. Sonochem.* **2009**, *16*, 63–69.
36. Rolich, T.; Rezić, I.; Ćurković, L. Estimation of Steel Guitar Strings Corrosion by Artificial Neural Network. *Corr. Sci.* **2010**, *52*, 996–1002.
37. Rezić, I.; Steffan, I. ICP-OES determination of metals present in textile materials. *Microchem. J.* **2007**, *85*, 46–51.
38. Rezić, I.; Ćurković, L.; Ujević, M. Simple methods for characterization of metals in historical textile threads. *Talanta* **2010**, *82*, 237–244.
39. Rezić, I.; Špehar, M.; Jakovljević, S. Characterization of Ag and Au nanolayers on Cu alloys by TLC, SEM-EDS, and ICP-OES. *Mater. Corr.* **2017**, *68*, 560–565.
40. Rezić, I.; Zeiner, M.; Steffan, I. Determination of 28 selected elements in textiles by axially viewed inductively coupled plasma optical emission spectrometry. *Talanta* **2011**, *83*, 865–871.
41. Reza Mahdavi, S.; Talesh, T.A. The effect of ultrasonic irradiation on the structure, morphology and photocatalytic performance of ZnO nanoparticles by sol-gel method. *Ultrason. Sonochem.* **2017**, *39*, 504–510.
42. Pokrovac, I,; Antimicrobial effect of colloidal nanopartcles of metals and metal oxides on MRSA and MSSA (in Croatian), University of Zagreb, Faculty of Pharmacy and biochemistry, Master's Thesis, 2018, September (Mentors prof. I. Kosalec and prof. I. Rezić);

https://repozitorij.pharma.unizg.hr/islandora/object/pharma:1100/datastream/PDF/download (accessed on January 2021).
43. Rezić, I.; Kiš, A.; Design of Experiment Approach to Optimize Hydrophobic Fabric Treatments. *Polymers*, **2020**, *09*, 2-15.
44. Li W.R., Xie X.B., Shi Q.S., Duan S.S., Ouyang Y.S., Chen Y.B. Antibacterial effect of silver nanoparticles on *Staphylococcus aureus. Biometals* **2011,** *24*, 135-141.
45. Mirzajani F., Ghassempour A., Aliahmadi A., Esmaeili M.A. Antibacterial effect of silver nanoparticles on *Staphylococcus aureus. Res Microbiol* **2011,** *162,* 542-549.
46. Grigor'eva A., Saranina I., Tikunova N., Safonov A., Timoshenko N., Rebrov A., Ryabchikova E. Fine mechanisms of the interaction of silver nanoparticles with the cells of *Salmonella typhimurium* and *Staphylococcus aureus. Biometals.* **2013,** *26,* 479-488.
47. Martinaga Pintarić, L.; Somogy Škoc, M.; Ljoljić Bilić, V.; Pokrovac, I.; Kosalec, I.; Rezić, I. Synthesis, Modification and Characterization of Antimicrobial Textile Surface Containing ZnO Nanoparticles. *Polymers,* **2020**, *12.* 1210-15.
48. Moore T.L., Rodriguez-Lorenzo L., V. Hirsch, S. Balog, D. Urban, C. Jud, B. Rothen-Rutishauser, M. Lattuada. A. Petri-Fink, Nanoparticle colloidal stability in cell culture media and impact on cellular interactions. *Chem. Soc. Rev.*, **2015**, *44*, 6287-6305.
49. Panáček A., Kvítek L., Prucek R., Kolář M., Večeřová R., Pizúrová N., Zbořil R. Silver Colloid Nanoparticles: Synthesis, Characterization, and Their Antibacterial Activity. *J Phys Chem B*, **2006**, *110(33),* 16248–16253.
50. Ansari M., Khan H., Khan A., Sultan A., Azam A. Characterization of clinical strains of MSSA, MRSA and MRSE isolated from skin and soft tissue infections and the antibacterial activity of ZnO nanoparticles. *World J Microb Biot*, **2012**, *28*, 1605-1613.

CHAPTER FIVE

ANTIMICROBIAL MICROCAPSULES[1]

Introduction

The significance of polymers in combating microbial resistant strains has captured the attention of engineers. This attention stems from the potential of silver ions and silver nanoparticles to amplify the antimicrobial attributes of microcapsules. These microcapsules serve as vehicles for controlled substance release, thereby extending the duration of antimicrobial efficacy. The primary objective of this study was to impart antimicrobial functionality to diverse polymer surfaces through the integration of core/shell microcapsules endowed with antimicrobial silver. The construction of these microcapsules involved a sodium alginate shell encapsulating antimicrobial silver in the core, which were subsequently applied to polymer surfaces using the dip-coating technique. A comprehensive analysis of the functionalized polymers ensued, employing an array of spectroscopic and microscopic methods. Through meticulous characterization before and after functionalization, the temporal release of active agents was closely monitored. The culmination of these efforts furnishes valuable insights into determining the optimal concentration of antimicrobial silver required for encapsulation, ensuring the desired sustained release profiles are achieved.

> Antimicrobial agents can be preserved until they reach the targeted bacteria in different forms. If they are encapsulated, their release can be guided in time and in direction that is the most suitable for the antimicrobial treatment.

[1] I. Rezić, M. Somogyi Škoc, M. Majdak, S. Jurić, K. Sopko Stracenski, M. Vinceković, Functionalization of Polymer Surface with Antimicrobial Microcapsules, Polymers 14 (2022) 1961, doi.org/10.3390/ polym14101961

Encapsulation

The effectiveness of antimicrobial coatings hinges on the size of nanoparticles, which are notably smaller than bacteria. This size discrepancy is pivotal for achieving optimal penetration through bacterial cell walls, thereby inducing impactful effects on microorganisms [1,2]. Silver, renowned for its potent antimicrobial properties [3–6], serves as a key agent in this endeavour. The modification of polymer surfaces entails a gamut of characterization techniques [7–13], prominently featuring various spectroscopic methodologies [14–18]. Moreover, for efficient sample preparation and analysis of specific metal ions, liquid or ion chromatography assumes significance [19–23]. However, complex samples like encapsulated nanoparticles necessitate a fusion of diverse methodologies.

While microencapsulation technology's roots trace back to the 1940s, the past decade has witnessed widespread utilization of encapsulated products across diverse industries such as agriculture, food, cosmetics, and textiles. Particularly in the medical realm, microencapsulated materials have gained traction due to their capacity for prolonged release of active compounds [3]. Microencapsulation involves ensconcing small particles with a desired coating, yielding diameters typically spanning 2 to 2000 μm. Wall thickness averages 0.5–150 μm, with core composition ranging from 20 to 95% of total weight. The encapsulation method employed hinges on the intended purpose of the microcapsules.

Microencapsulation offers a gamut of benefits, prominently including safeguarding active agents, controlled release, facile handling, and targeted delivery. Various encapsulation techniques exist, encompassing both physical processes (e.g., air suspension coating, coextrusion, rotating disk atomization, spray drying, spray cooling) and chemical methods (e.g., matrix polymerization, liposome technology, coacervation, solvent extraction, solvent evaporation). Coacervation, a technique within the latter category, yields core–shell microcapsules via interactions between oppositely charged polyelectrolytes in aqueous media. Noteworthy attributes of coacervation encompass high payload, encapsulation efficiency surpassing 99%, cost-effectiveness, and compatibility with ambient conditions [24]. This process entails electrostatic interactions between two aqueous phases.

A diverse array of hydrophilic polymers, including sodium alginate, gelatine, and chitosan, finds common application in crafting polymeric micro- or nano-capsules [25]. Coacervation, a well-established technique, employs phase separation to generate two distinct liquid phases. The initial phase comprises a polymer-rich coacervate, while the second phase consists of a polymer-depleted equilibrium solution. This coacervation process accommodates both polar and non-polar species. In more intricate coacervation setups, the encapsulation of active agents involves the combination of two distinct species, such as gelatine and gum Arabic, or sodium alginate and chitosan [26]. Chitosan, insoluble in alkaline pH environments, precipitates upon contact with an alkaline solution. This reaction involves introducing chitosan into an alkali solution via a compressed air nozzle, resulting in particle formation. Subsequently, the encapsulated particles are separated through filtration [27].

Coacervation stands as one of the earliest and most prevalent microencapsulation methods. Depending on the procedure, it can be categorized into simple coacervation, where colloidal substances like gelatine or chitosan are employed, and complex coacervation, which entails preparing a polymeric solution from two oppositely charged colloids. Examples of the latter include gelatine with gum Arabic or chitosan in combination [28]. (Table 5.1) [28].

Table 5.1. Shell and core materials used in coacervation

Coacervation		
Polymer	**Coacervation Agent**	**Nanoparticle**
Chitosan	NaOH	Silver

Once antimicrobial microcapsules laden with silver active agents have been created, the subsequent challenge lies in affixing these microcapsules onto the surface of polymer materials [28, 29, 30, 31]. In this context, the dip-coating immersion process emerges as an ideal solution. This technique involves immersing the substrate into a liquid solution and subsequently withdrawing it at a controlled speed, under specific temperature and atmospheric conditions. The liquid medium contains the antimicrobial components [32, 33, 34]. A recent area of emphasis pertains to the utilization of gold or silver nanoparticles [35, 36, 37]. Effective characterization of such materials necessitates a judicious amalgamation of spectroscopic and microscopic methodologies [38, 39, 40].

The dip-coating process encompasses three distinct stages. Firstly, the substrate is immersed into the liquid solution. Subsequently, a wet layer is formed on the substrate. Finally, the coating is dried through solvent evaporation [41].

This multistep procedure culminates in the successful integration of antimicrobial microcapsules onto the polymer material's surface, facilitating enhanced antimicrobial functionality and applications [42].

The immersion process unfolds deliberately, affording ample time for the coating to align into a more advantageous and compact arrangement. Careful solvent evaporation is essential to avoid destabilization, with the concurrent occurrence of cross-linking leading to heightened rigidity and heat-induced fusion of the resulting gel. This coagulation temperature is contingent upon the specific composition [41, 42, 43]. Diverse factors exert influence on film outcome and thickness during immersion, encompassing parameters like salt viscosity, surface tension, and pressure. Optimization of these parameters underscores the proficient adherence of microcapsules to the polymer surface, concurrently elevating the antimicrobial impact, especially with the integration of silver nanoparticles [44, 45, 46]. Colloidal nanoparticles confer numerous advantages [47, 48, 49, 50], necessitating intricate characterization techniques [51, 52].

The core of these microcapsules harbours antimicrobial silver, with Pandey et al.'s notable work revealing that the method of silver nanoparticle stabilization significantly modulates antimicrobial efficacy. Impressively, silver nanoparticles exhibited pronounced bactericidal potency surpassing their effects on fungi and other microorganisms [6], thereby highlighting their broad antibacterial potential [7–11]. Fostering adhesion between encapsulated active agents and polymer surfaces is achieved through dip-coating methodology, employing the sol–gel binding mechanism to anchor microcapsules onto textile carriers [53, 54, 55, 56]. The well-established sol-gel technique, renowned for generating uniform coatings, is especially suited for conferring antimicrobial protection [57].

Endowed with versatile properties, microcapsules find utility across diverse industries [58]. Consequently, considerable research is dedicated to formulating applications for healthcare, particularly within textiles [59, 60]. This study revolves around the functionalization of polymer surfaces through antimicrobial silver-loaded microcapsules. The innovation lies in circumventing the traditional route of direct nanoparticle functionalization, opting instead for shell/core microcapsules encapsulating antimicrobial silver compounds. This encapsulation strategy facilitates timed release, thereby augmenting the polymer's antimicrobial potency. The research hones the microencapsulation process, sequentially leveraging simple and complex coacervation steps to enhance subsequent polymer functionalization by dip-coating methodology.

The main hypotheses driving our research are as follows: (*i*) the synthesis of antimicrobial microcapsules, varying in size and chemical composition with antimicrobial silver, is feasible; (*ii*) facile application of these microcapsules onto polymer surfaces can be achieved through dip-coating methodology; and (*iii*) the resultant novel materials, embedded with microcapsules, exhibit controlled Ag release over time, rendering them suitable for medical applications. Throughout this study, reagents of utmost purity were employed, including dithizone, 1,5-diphenylthiocarbazone ($C_{13}H_{12}N_4S$) from Merck (Darmstadt, Germany), 96% ethanol (C_2H_5OH) from Gram-Mol (Zagreb, Croatia), silver nitrate ($AgNO_3$) from Gram-Mol (Croatia), zinc sulphate 7-hydrate ($ZnSO_4 \times 7H_2O$) from Gram-Mol (Zagreb, Croatia), and 3-glycidyloxypropyltrimethoxysilane (GLYMO, 98%) from Aldrich Chemicals. For testing purposes, sodium alginate ($C_6H_9NaO_7$) from Sigma-Aldrich was utilized. Spectroscopic analysis was carried out using a two-beam UV/VIS Lambda 20 spectrometer from Perkin Elmer (Waltham, MA, USA) with measurements performed in 10 mm quartz cuvettes also from Perkin Elmer. In this study, the encapsulation process of silver-filled microcapsule samples was achieved through a reaction involving the interaction of polymer anions with polyvalent cations, resulting in the formation of an outer shell.

This process was primarily facilitated by the external ionotropic method, and its procedural steps are outlined in Figure 1: (1) polymer droplets containing an active ingredient were immersed in a homogeneous solution containing the crosslinker; (2) interaction between the crosslinker and polymer occurred; (3) subsequent formation of the outer shell took place [28]. The encapsulation procedure was carried out under specific conditions, including a pressure of 530 mbar, an amplitude of 5, a frequency of 2000 Hz, and heating at 50°C. During encapsulation, solution droplets precipitated into the zinc sulphate 7-hydrate solution. Upon completion, the resulting microcapsules underwent 60 minutes of stirring, followed by filtration and subsequent washing with distilled water. The resultant microcapsules exhibited a core replete with silver ions, encased within a shell composed of sodium alginate and zinc sulphate 7-hydrate.

For the encapsulation process, the initial step involved preparing a solution of sodium alginate with a concentration of 1.5%. Simultaneously, a solution of zinc sulphate 7-hydrate was concocted with a concentration of 1M. To create the 1.5% sodium alginate solution, 7.50 g of sodium alginate was dissolved in a 500 mL volumetric flask using distilled water. The encapsulation process employed here utilized simple coacervation within sodium alginate samples containing zinc sulphate 7-hydrate in the outer shell. Encapsulation involves phase separation of a macromolecular solution into two immiscible liquid phases: a denser coacervate phase and a diluted equilibrium solution.

The process encompasses four key stages depicted in Figure 1: (1) dispersion of the active substance into a solution of a surface-active colloid;

(2) precipitation of the colloid onto dispersed droplets; (3) introduction of a second colloid to trigger polymer–polymer complex coacervation; and (4) stabilization through the addition of chitosan, a cross-linking agent (Figure 5.1) [28].

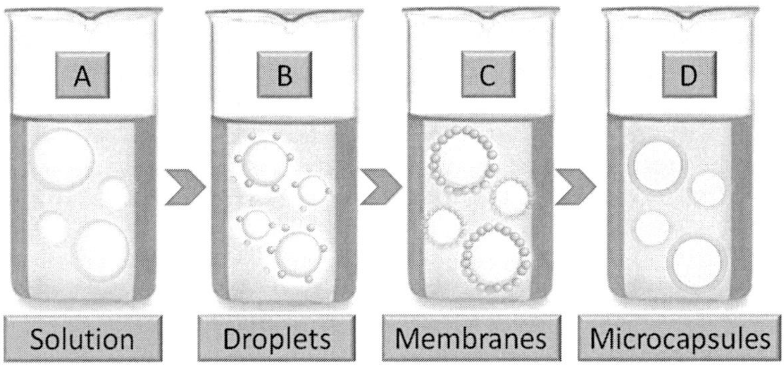

Figure 5.1. Phases in the encapsulation process

For the preparation of zinc sulphate 7-hydrate, 143.77 g was weighed and added to a 500 mL volumetric flask, followed by the addition of water to reach the mark. The flask contents were thoroughly shaken to ensure proper mixing. Subsequently, a solution of sodium alginate and $AgNO_3$ was generated. This involved dissolving 0.0332 g of $AgNO_3$ in 100 mL of sodium alginate solution, which was stirred using a magnetic stirrer for 30 minutes. The resulting solution underwent vacuum filtration to remove impurities. Before initiating the encapsulation procedure, a 100 mL zinc sulphate 7-hydrate solution was placed in a 600 mL beaker, serving as the solidifying agent during encapsulation. Simultaneously, 100 mL of the filtered solution was poured into a 500 mL bottle. Nitrogen pressure was employed to propel the solution through a silicone tube, culminating at a 20 μm diameter nozzle. En route to the nozzle, the solution encountered a heater to prevent clotting. A magnetic vibrator was utilized to encourage microcapsule formation, and the encapsulated setup.

Throughout encapsulation, solution droplets descended into the zinc sulphate 7-hydrate solution for solidification. Post-encapsulation, the microcapsules were stirred for 60 minutes to ensure thorough solidification. Following this, they were filtered, washed with distilled water, and stored in a cool, dark environment.

The resulting microcapsules boasted a core comprised of $AgNO_3$, ensconced within a shell of zinc sulphate 7-hydrate. The microcapsules exhibited a purple hue due to staining caused by the presence of $AgNO_3$.

Subsequently, a subset of the microcapsules was dispersed in a chitosan solution (0.5% CS in 1.0% CH_3COOH) under constant magnetic stirring for approximately 30 minutes. This facilitated the formation of a chitosan layer around the microcapsules, contributing to their structure. After this step, the microcapsules were again filtered, rinsed, and stored in a cool, dark location prior to further characterization. Furthermore, several microcapsules were allowed to air-dry at room temperature until reaching their equilibrium moisture content.

> Encapsulation can be used for preserving not only nanoparticles and inorganic materials, but also organic antimicrobial agents, such are for example oils, resins and other liquid forms of substances.

The release of the active substance, Ag+ cations, from the microcapsules occurs through diffusion. To initiate diffusion testing, approximately 1 ± 0.0001 g of microcapsules were accurately weighed into a 100 mL beaker using random sampling. Following this, 20 mL of distilled water was added using a pipette. A total of 23 aqueous solutions were prepared using this method for subsequent testing. The solutions were then agitated under the following conditions: default shaking speed 4 (out of 10 possible speeds), shaking time 60 min, and no heating.

After the 60-minute agitation period, the solutions were filtered to separate the microcapsules from the solution, as microcapsules could interfere with spectrometric analysis. To quantify the concentration of Ag+ cation and monitor the analysis, a calibration curve, or calibration diagram, was essential. Quantitative and qualitative analysis was carried out using a two-beam UV/VIS Lambda 20 spectrometer in the UV and visible range, covering wavelengths from 190 to 900 nm. Quartz cuvettes were employed for UV range testing.

Prior to testing, the dithizone solution needed to be diluted 1:9 with distilled water in a 10 mL volumetric flask. Since the microcapsules contain zinc sulphate 7-hydrate, which could potentially interfere with silver determination, the standard addition method was employed to mitigate this interference. This method involves adding a standard solution of known concentration to the test solution. To create a coloured complex for spectroscopic investigation, dithizone, which dissolves in carbon tetrachloride, chloroform, and 96% ethanol, was utilized [61].

To avoid toxic chemicals, a 0.07% dithizone solution was used for testing, requiring filtration before use to eliminate residual dithizone. It's important to note that dithizone itself reacts non-selectively with all metals present in the test solution [63]. To create the calibration curve, a triton of

$AgNO_3$ with a concentration of 0.1 M was employed as a standard solution. Standard solutions were mixed with dithizone in a 1:1 volume ratio and transferred to 25 mL volumetric flasks, yielding a highly correlated set of calculated absorbances.

Furthermore, a TLC (Thin-Layer Chromatography) method was developed for analysing metal ions extractable from the microcapsules. Extensive experimentation with over 30 stationary phases and different mobile phase compositions, including optimal solvent mixtures containing hydrochloric acid and water, led to the chromatographic method employing ACN (acetonitrile), HCl (hydrochloric acid), and H_2O (water) in a 60.00:19.17:20.83 v/v% ratio, respectively.

Fixing encapsulated nanoparticles

The dip-coating process was meticulously executed in the following manner: Firstly, the sol was magnetically stirred to achieve the optimal molar ratio of 3-glycidyloxypropyltrimethoxysilane (GLYMO) to water, a parameter that was fine-tuned based on previous experience to ensure the retention of textile attributes such as softness and hand value [42,47,55]. The sol-gel properties were influenced by a range of critical parameters such as the precursor, catalyst types, solvent, precursor-to-solvent molar ratio, pH value, and temperature, all tailored to the physical and chemical characteristics of the chosen GLYMO precursor and HCl catalyst.

Secondly, a solution of distilled water and ethanol was meticulously mixed to allow for the removal of volatile substances through evaporation before or during condensation. Subsequently, GLYMO was added and the solution was stirred continuously using a magnetic stirrer until homogeneity was achieved. Thirdly, samples were cut to dimensions of 5 × 5 cm^2 to facilitate the dip-coating process on a custom-made apparatus at a predetermined drawing speed of 1 mm/s. Lastly, the modified samples were left to gel at room temperature for 24 hours and then subjected to drying at 100 °C for 1 hour. In the case of antimicrobial treatment, silver ions from silver nitrate were methodically introduced to the sol in small, careful amounts under higher mixing speed, ensuring the formation of a homogeneous solution.

The detailed procedure for surface modification via the sol-gel method was optimized in prior work, involving the functionalization of polymers using 3-glycidyloxypropyltrimethoxysilane (GLYMO). Nanoparticles within microcapsules underwent gelation at room temperature followed by heating at 100 °C for 60 minutes. The modified products underwent characterization via various instrumental techniques, including thin layer chromatography (TLC), scanning electron microscopy with an energy-dispersive X-ray (EDX) detector (SEM-EDX), and Fourier-transform infrared (FTIR) spectroscopy utilizing attenuated total reflectance (ATR) techniques [47]. While the earlier work focused on modification using microcapsules filled with different compounds, the present study showcases the outcomes of microcapsules filled with silver compounds, particularly emphasizing their antimicrobial properties.

Several crucial factors influenced the efficacy of the functionalization process, such as the speed of immersion, concentration, viscosity of solutions, surface tension, and sample dimensions. Dip coating was applied to both woven and nonwoven polymers, with the molar ratio of GLYMO to water playing a pivotal role, determined through experimental results. An optimal ratio was identified based on desired outcomes, such as uniform distribution of antibacterial silver, smooth texture, optimal shine, and flexibility to withstand forces without cracking.

The composition of the sample, determined according to the ISO 1833.22 standard norm procedure, involved cellulose fibres with a mass per unit ascertained using ISO 2286-2 as 186.7 g/m^2. No preliminary treatment of the textile substrate (scouring, bleaching, etc.) was conducted prior to dip coating.

FTIR characterization of polymers functionalized with antimicrobial microcapsules was carried out using a Fourier-transform infrared spectrometer (Spectrum 100 FTIR, Perkin Elmer) employing KBr and ATR techniques. Spectra were recorded in a frequency range from 400 to 4000 cm^-1 in diffuse reflectance mode, at a resolution of 4 cm^{-1}. This specific configuration enabled the collection of solid-state spectra of the samples.

The findings of this study mark a significant stride towards addressing the challenge of antimicrobial-resistant microorganisms. Microencapsulation proves intriguing as it facilitates controlled release of antimicrobial agents, is adaptable to various materials without altering the original polymer, and boasts a valid shelf life. The core compound of all prepared microcapsules in this investigation was the antibacterial silver ion, offering a promising avenue to combatting powerful resistant microorganisms.

The selection of this material was driven by its well-established potent antimicrobial properties against a broad spectrum of bacteria, encompassing both Gram-positive and Gram-negative strains, including those that are resistant to antibiotics. The application of encapsulation methods further amplifies the utility of antimicrobial silver. The controlled release capability of microcapsules has opened avenues for potential storage, stabilization, and deployment in various products. Within this study, microcapsules were synthesized to serve as antimicrobial agents tailored for medical applications. These applications span a range of uses such as wound dressings, materials for treating wounds, hospital bedding, and similar contexts. The decision to utilize antimicrobial silver was underpinned by existing literature references and empirical assessments. Our prior investigations also encompassed antimicrobial assessment of silver nanoparticles, with a focus on their activity against the model microorganism *S. aureus*.

Figure 5.2 visually represents the microcapsules crafted through the simple coacervation process. These microcapsules are laden with silver ions within their core, encapsulated by an alginate shell infused with zinc sulphate 7 hydrate.

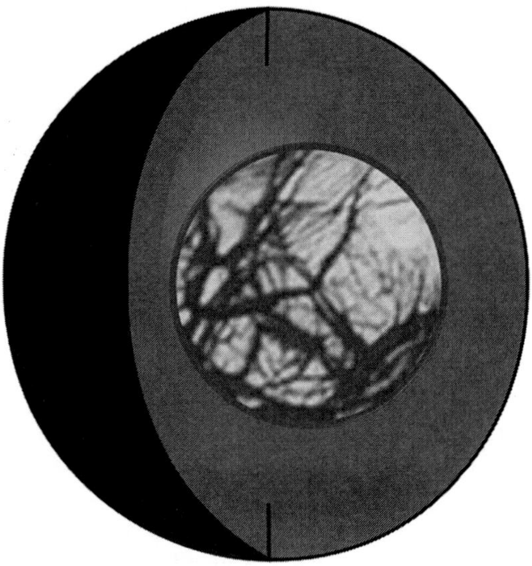

Figure 5.2. Shematic overview of microcapsules filled with silver ion of 450 μm in diameter

Additionally, a subset of microcapsules underwent further encapsulation by the addition of chitosan during the complete coacervation process. It is important to emphasize that no alterations were made to any physical, chemical, or morphological property of the antimicrobial silver filling within the microcapsules during their production. The primary goal was to maintain the integrity of the modification and functionalization steps on the polymer surface without introducing any differences to the final microcapsule product.

After capturing microphotographs of the encapsulated microcapsules using high-resolution optical microscopy, a scanning electron microscope (SEM) was employed to ascertain the dimensions of the pores and shells of the individual microcapsules following lyophilization. The combination of these techniques is a widely utilized approach for the comprehensive characterization of microcapsules. The SEM results are visually depicted in Figure 3A. Analysis of this figure reveals that the average diameter of the microcapsules ranged from 140 to 285 μm in diameter. By comparing these results with those presented in Figure 2, it becomes evident that the reduction in microcapsule size after lyophilization was in the range of 37% to 69%. Notably, a critical observation was the absence of cracks in the microcapsules after the lyophilization process.

This observation substantiates that the lyophilization process was appropriately executed, without causing any detriment to the microcapsule shell. Similar findings were reported by Glaucia et al., 2013 [56], who discussed the importance of these attributes in ensuring enhanced protection and retention of the encapsulated material. Their research involving the encapsulation of sucralose through double emulsion followed by complex coacervation revealed that solid bridges resulting from the lyophilization process contributed to the clustering of microcapsules [56].

Furthermore, their conclusions aligned with ours, demonstrating that the average particle size remained unaffected by variations in the shell material. Nevertheless, Glaucia et al. noted that the concentration of the encapsulating agent did exert an influence on the average particle size [56]. In contrast, He et al. [57] employed spray drying, rather than lyophilization, for the microcapsules prior to SEM investigation.

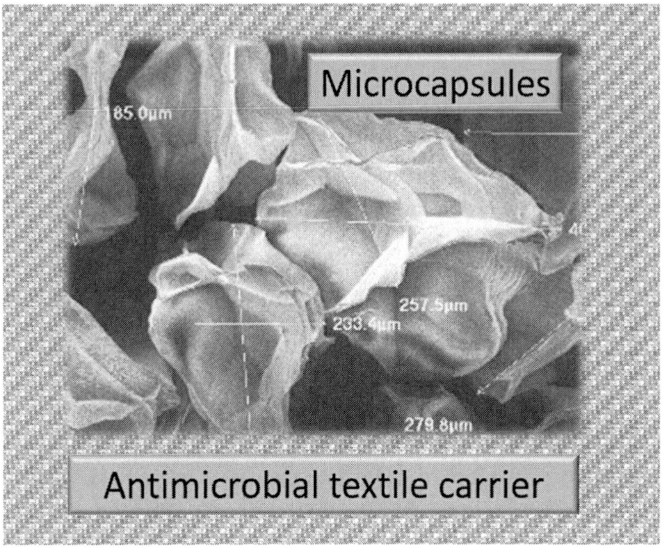

Figure 5.3. Antimicrobial textile carrier with microcapsules

He et al.'s findings indicated a broader distribution of particle sizes for spray-dried microcapsules, spanning the range of 1 to 100 µm, with the majority centered around 10–30 µm [57]. In contrast, our SEM results, presented in Figure 3A, reveal that the size of the microcapsules fell within the range of 150 to 400 nm, while the pore size among these microcapsules was between 50 to 100 nm.

The SEM-EDX results, as depicted in Figure 5.4, confirm the presence of both zinc and silver within the microcapsules. To probe the release of silver from the microcapsule core, further investigation was undertaken through chromatographic screening and quantitative UV-VIS spectroscopy.

For qualitative identification of silver release from the microcapsules, thin-layer chromatography was employed. The chromatographic method allows for the tracking of silver among other metals due to its distinctive retention factor (RF) value. In our chromatographic system, with a composition of ACN: HCl: H2O in a 60.00: 19.17: 20.83 v/v% ratio, silver was detectable using various indicators (refer to Table 5.2).

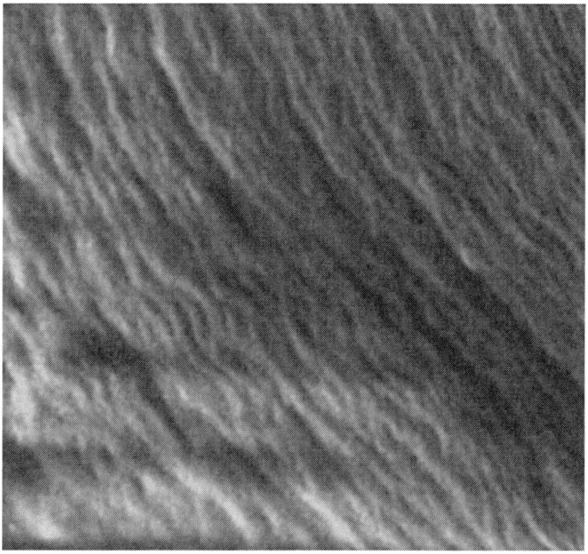

Figure 5.4. SEM-EDX chemical characterization of the surface of microcapsules

The UV-VIS spectroscopic characterization was carried out within the wavelength range of 400 to 600 nm. Figure 5A illustrates the UV-VIS curves acquired during the investigation, while Figure 5B depicts the corresponding calibration curve derived from the obtained results. The calibration curve was generated employing five AgNO3 solutions of known concentrations.

Table 5.2. Thin-layer chromatography data

Detection of Silver through Its R_F Value and Characteristic Colours			
Without Indicator	**Dimethylglioxime**	**Quercetin**	**Alizarin Red S**
+	+	+	+ Zn pink spot

Standardized preparation was employed for all samples: initially, 1 mL of dithizone was introduced into five 25 mL volumetric flasks containing AgNO3 solutions. Subsequently, an equivalent volume of dithizone to that of AgNO3 solutions was added to each sample. The absorption measurements were conducted at a maximum wavelength of 512 nm, and the recorded absorption values are presented in Figure 5.5.

Before delving into the analysis of silver release from the antimicrobial microcapsules, an essential preliminary step was the determination of the samples. The calibration curve depicted in Figure 5B was utilized to ascertain the silver release (as shown in Figure 5.5). During the diffusion process in an aqueous medium, Ag+ cations migrate from the microcapsules into the surrounding medium.

The diffusion process itself is graphically depicted in Figure 5C, alongside the resultant spectral curves. The quantitative assessment of silver content in microcapsules with varying diameters (120 μm or 450 μm) revealed silver concentrations ranging from 100 to 350 μg/g, respectively. These concentrations hold significance, particularly in the context of medical materials intended for protective applications

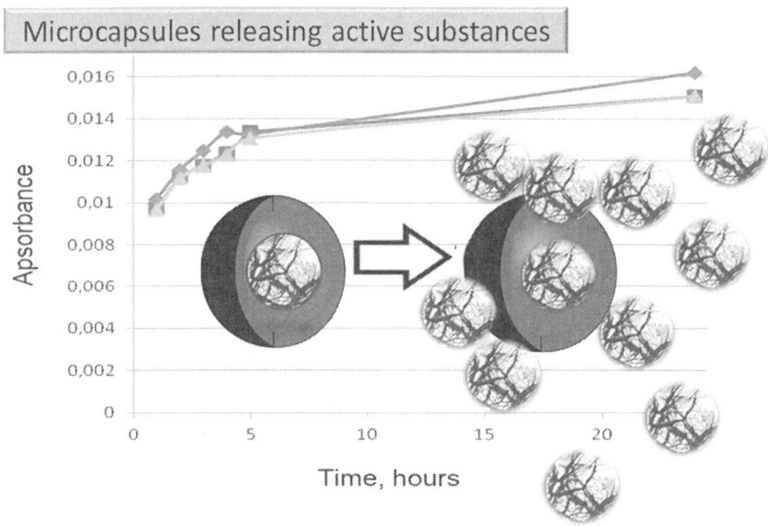

Figure 5.5. UV-VIS data of the active substances release over 24 h from microcapsules

Figure 5.6. presents the microphotograph of the samples (woven and non-woven cotton and viscose polymers), before and after the modification

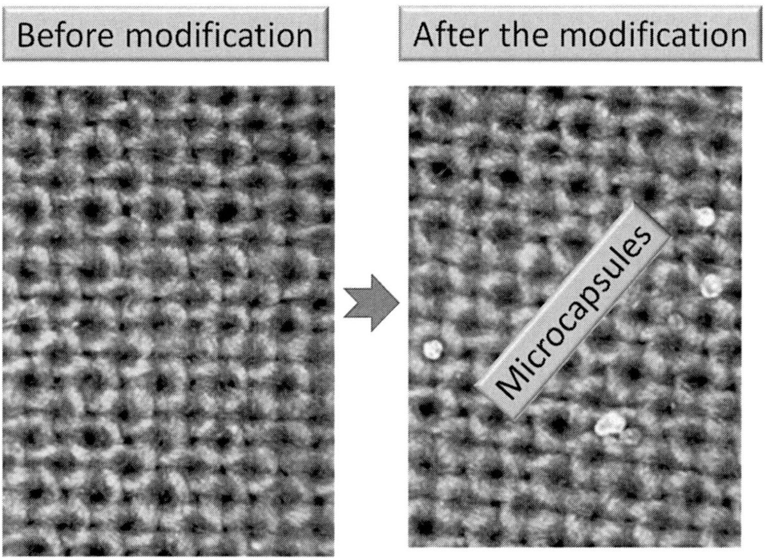

Figure 5.6. Microphotograph of the samples before and after the modification with microcapsules[5]

For the spectroscopic analysis of the samples, Fourier-transform infrared spectrometry (FTIR) was employed using the Spectrum 100 FTIR instrument from Perkin Elmer, Waltham, Massachusetts. The resulting FTIR spectrum is presented in Figure 6. Subsequently, the newly prepared microcapsules underwent impregnation through a dip-coating process onto various substrates, including 100% viscose nonwoven fabric, woven viscose, and viscose/cellulose polymers. As depicted in Figure 5.3, the progress of the dip-coating process can be monitored through the formation of specific functional groups that emerge during the sol-gel procedure. Attenuated Total Reflectance Fourier-transform infrared spectroscopy (ATR-FTIR) is a valuable analytical technique that permits the analysis of microcapsules without intricate sample preparation, thereby increasing analysis speed and sample throughput.

ATR-FTIR is particularly advantageous in determining the shell thickness of antimicrobial microcapsules, as it can penetrate into the micro meter range, offering insights into the character of functional groups present in the microcapsule shells.

The research focused on the development of microcapsules as carriers of antimicrobial agents, with specific emphasis on antimicrobial silver. Previous investigations have highlighted the potent antimicrobial effects of small silver nanoparticles against various microorganisms, including bacteria and fungi. Furthermore, these nanoparticles exhibited activity against drug-resistant strains of bacteria.

In this study, the antibacterial efficacy of the antimicrobial polymer coated with microcapsules was grounded in prior research on the antimicrobial effects of silver, which indicated maximal efficiency after 6 hours of exposure. Consequently, the concentrations used in this research were chosen based on the parameters associated with the peak antimicrobial efficiency of silver. The primary application envisaged for these materials was in potential bandages and wound care products.

The substantial potential of these newly developed materials is attributed to their functionalization, as evidenced by figures and tables, and notably, the FTIR-ATR spectra of the modified samples. The efficient application of antibacterial microcapsules onto the polymer surface, laden with antimicrobial silver, was successfully achieved.

The results of this investigation suggest that surfaces treated with such microcapsules may possess antimicrobial properties due to the presence of silver particles. However, further studies are warranted to delve deeper into this aspect.

Previous chapters and papers have consistently highlighted the strong antimicrobial properties of silver, particularly in nanoparticle form. For instance, nanoparticles with a size of 10 nm exhibited potent antimicrobial effects against Staphylococcus aureus in previous research. The work of Özyildiz and colleagues also aligns with the literature, where they developed antimicrobial textiles using encapsulated ozonated red pepper seed oil. These textiles exhibited significant antimicrobial properties against various microorganisms.

To comprehensively compare microcapsules produced through different approaches—simple and complex coacervation—further investigations are necessary, which will be the primary focus of next forthcoming research endeavours.

In contrast to our own research, Ramya and Maheshwari [54] employed microcapsules containing piper betel leaf extracts encapsulated within them. Their study involved fabrics made from a blend of 50:50% (W/W) cotton and bamboo fibres, and they applied microcapsules using the exhaustion method. They used spray encapsulation with calcium chloride and sodium alginate for encapsulation. Their findings indicated that the resulting textile material possessed antimicrobial properties effective against bacterial species commonly found in foot wounds, including Staphylococcus, Bacillus, Klebsiella, Pseudomonas, and Proteus. The materials treated with microcapsules exhibited superior results, particularly after washing.

The antibacterial activity and mechanism of silver against S. aureus strain ATCC 6538P was investigated by Li et al. [44], who determined that the minimal bactericidal concentration (MBC) was 20 μg/mL. These results can be compared with the findings of Mirzajani et al. [45], who demonstrated that 4 μg/mL of silver completely inhibited bacterial growth. Grigoreva et al. [46] also confirmed this interaction. Additionally, Shevtsova et al. [58] incorporated antimicrobial silver nanoparticles within temperature-responsive hybrid nanomaterials, resulting in significant improvements in antimicrobial application. Raczkowska et al. [59] presented "smart" antibacterial surfaces based on silver nanoparticles embedded in temperature-responsive coatings, demonstrating a temperature-switched killing effect against Escherichia coli and Staphylococcus aureus.

Konnova et al. reported a straightforward procedure for fabricating 50 nm silver nanoparticles and applying them against yeast and bacteria. They utilized cationic polymer-stabilized nanoparticles adhered to microbial cells, resulting in efficient delivery of silver nanoparticles into microorganisms. This concept of functionalizing biological cells with nanomaterials holds promise for various applications.

Given the increasing resistance of harmful bacteria to conventional drugs, the need for novel solutions and formulations to suppress bacterial growth on medical textiles is evident. Encapsulation, as explored in this study, presents a compelling technique for achieving controlled release of antimicrobial agents. The research successfully produced microcapsules (120 and 450 μm) composed of sodium alginate and zinc sulphate 7-hydrate, filled with silver, and characterized them using various microscopic and spectrometric methods. These microcapsules were effectively adhered to the surface of woven and nonwoven polymers (composed of viscose and cellulose) for the preparation of antimicrobial materials.

Furthermore, the release of active antimicrobial silver from the microcapsules was tracked over 25 hours in an aqueous medium to assess their potential as fillers for medical materials such as bandages and wound dressings.

The research findings confirm the main hypotheses of the study: (i) successful preparation of antimicrobial microcapsules with varying sizes and compositions; (ii) efficient application of microcapsules to polymer surfaces through dip-coating; and (iii) demonstrated release of antimicrobial silver from microcapsules, establishing their potential use in medical materials. Overall, these results indicate that the antimicrobial efficiency of these materials could inhibit the growth of specific microorganisms on open wounds.

References

1. World Health Organization. Antimicrobial Resistance Global Report on Surveillance 2014. Available online: https//www.who.int/drugresistance/documents/surveillancereport/en/ (accessed on 7 January 2020).
2. Van Kourtis, A.P.; Hatfield, K.; Baggs, J.; Mu, Y.; See, I.; Epson, E.; Nadle, J.; Kainer, M.A.; Dumyati, G.; Petit, S.; et al. Vital Signs: Epidemiology and Recent Trends in Methicillin-Resistant and in Methicillin-Susceptible *Staphylococcus aureus* Bloodstream Infections—United States. *Morb. Mortal. Wkly. Rep.* **2019**, *68*, 214–219.
3. Kirin, P. The Analysis of Antimicrobial Surface by Thin Layer Chromatography. Master's Thesis, University of Zagreb, Faculty of Textile Technology, Prilaz baruna Filipovića 28a 10000 Zagreb, Croatia, 2019.
4. Delaney, J.A.; Schneider-Lindner, V.; Brassard, P.; Suissa, S. Mortality after infection with methicillin-resistant *Staphylococcus aureus* (MRSA) diagnosed in the community. *BMC Med.* **2008**, *6*, 2.
5. Padmavathy, N.; Vijayaraghavan, R. Enhanced bioactivity of ZnO nanoparticles-an antimicrobial study. *Sci. Technol. Adv. Mater.* **2008**, *9*, 035004.
6. Pandey, S.; De Klerk, C.; Kim, J.; Kang, M.; Fosso-Kankeu, E. Eco Friendly Approach for Synthesis, Characterization and Biological Activities of Milk Protein Stabilized Silver Nanoparticles. *Polymers* **2020**, *12*, 1418. https://doi.org/10.3390/polym 12061418.
7. Pandey, S.; Ramontja, J. Sodium alginate stabilized silver nanoparticles-silica nanohybrid and their antibacterial characteristics. *Int. J. Biol. Macromol.* **2016**, *93*, 712–723.
8. Beyth, N.; Houri-Haddad, Y.; Domb, A.; Khan, W.; Hazan, R. Alternative Antimicrobial Approach Nano-Antimicrobial Materials. *Complement. Altern. Med.* **2015**, *2015*, 246012.
9. Dizaj, S.M.; Lotpoura, F.; Barzegar-Jalali, M.; Zarrintana, M.H.; Adibkiab, K. Antimicrobial activity of the metals and metal oxide nanoparticles. *Mater. Sci. Eng. C* **2014**, *44*, 278–284.
10. Emami-Karvani, Z.; Chehrazi, P. Antibacterial activity of ZnO nanoparticle on Gram-positive and Gram-negative bacteria. *Afr. J. Microbiol. Res.* **2011**, *5*, 1368–1373.
11. Rasmussen, J.W.; Martinez, E.; Louka, P.; Wingett, D.G. Zinc oxide nanoparticles for selective destruction of tumor cells and potential for drug delivery applications. *Expert Opin. Drug Deliv.* **2010**, *7*, 1063–1077.

12. Rastin, H.; Ormsby, R.T.; Atkins, G.J.; Losic, D. 3D Bioprinting of Methylcellulose/Gelatin-Methacryloyl (MC/GelMA) Bioink with High Shape Integrity. *ACS Appl. Bio Mater.* **2020**, *3*, 1815–1826.
13. Peak, C.V.; Singh, K.A.; Adlouni, M.; Chen, J.; Gaharwar, A.K. Printing Therapeutic Proteins in 3D using Nanoengineered Bioink to Control and Direct Cell Migration, *Adv. Health Mater.* **2019**, *8*, e1801553.
14. Mohammad, J.; Hajipour, M.J.; Fromm, K.M.; Ashkarran, A.A.; Aberasturi, D.J.; Larramendi, I.R.; Rojo, T.; Serpooshan, V.; Parak, W.J.; Mahmoud, M. Erratum: Antibacterial properties of nanoparticles. *Trends Biotech.***2012**, *30*, 499–511.
15. Raghupathi, K.R.; Koodali, R.T.; Manna, A.C. Size-dependent bacterial growth inhibition and mechanism of antibacterial activity of zinc oxide nanoparticles. *Langmuir* **2011**, *27*, 4020–4028.
16. Varner, K. *State of the Science Literature Review: Everything Nanosilver and More*; Scientific, Technical, Research, Engineering and Modeling Support Final Report.; EPA/600/R-10/084; U.S. Environmental Protection Agency, Office of Research and Development: Washington, DC, USA, 2010; pp. 15–18.
17. Rastin, H.; Zhang, B.; Bi, J.; Hassan, K.; Tung, T.T.; Losic, D. 3D printing of cell-laden electroconductive bioinks for tissue engineering applications. *J. Mater. Chem. B* **2020**, *8*, 5862–5876.
18. Rastin, H.; Zhang, B.; Mazinani, A.; Hassan, K.; Bi, J.; Tung, T.T.; Losic, D. 3D bioprinting of cell-laden electroconductive MXene nanocomposite bioinks. *Nanoscale* **2020**, *12*, 16069–16080.
19. Abramova, A.V.; Abramova, V.O.; Bayazitova, V.M.; Voitova, Y.; Straumal, E.A.; Lermontov, S.A.; Cherdyntseva, T.A.; Braeutigam, P.; Weiße, M.; Günther, K. A sol-gel method for applying nanosized antibacterial particles to the surface of textile materials in an ultrasonic field. *Ultrason. Sonochem.* **2020**, *60*, 104788.
20. Akhavan, F.; Majid Montazer, S. In situ sonosynthesis of nano TiO_2 on cotton fabric. *Ultrason. Sonochem.* **2014**, *21*, 681–691.
21. Behzadnia, A.; Montazer, M.; MahmoudiRad, M. In situ photo sonosynthesis and characterize nonmetal/metal dual doped honeycomb-like ZnO nanocomposites on wool fabric. *Ultrason. Sonochem.* **2015**, *27*, 200–209.
22. Ahmadizadegan, H.; Esmaielzadeha, S.; Ranjbara, M.; Marzban, Z.; Ghavas, F. Synthesis and characterization of polyester bionanocomposite membrane with ultrasonic irradiation process for gas permeation and antibacterial activity. *Ultrason. Sonochem.* **2018**, *41*, 538–550.

23. Ghayempour, S.; Montazer, M. Ultrasound irradiation based *in-situ* synthesis of star-like *Tragacanth gum*/zinc oxide nanoparticles on cotton fabric. *Ultrason. Sonochem.* **2017**, *34*, 458–465.
24. Timilsena, Y.P.; Akanbi, T.O.; Khalid, N.; Adhikari, B.; Barrow, C.J. Complex coacervation: Principles, mechanisms and applications in microencapsulation. *Int. J. Biol. Macromol.* **2019**, *121*, 1276–1286.
25. Jana, S. Natural polymeric biodegradable nanoblend for macromolecules delivery. In *Recent Developments in Polymer Macro, Micro and Nano Blends*; Elsevier: Amsterdam, The Netherlands, 2017; pp. 289–312.
26. Chadha, S. Recent advances in nano-encapsulation technologies for controlled release of biostimulants and antimicrobial agents. In *Advances in Nano-Fertilizers and Nano-Pesticides in Agriculture*; Elsevier: Amsterdam, The Netherlands, 2021; pp. 111–146.
27. Giri, T.K. Nanoarchitectured Polysaccharide-Based Drug Carrier for Ocular Therapeutics. In *Nanoarchitectonics for Smart Delivery and Drug Targeting*; Elsevier: Amsterdam, The Netherlands, 2016; pp. 29–55.
28. Salaün, F. Microencapsulation technology for smart textile coatings. In *Textiles, Active Coatings for Smart Textiles*; Woodhead Publishing Series; Elsevier: Amsterdam, The Netherlands, 2016; pp. 179–220.
29. Yadav, A.; Prasad, V.; Kathe, A.A.; Raj, S.; Yadav, D.; Sundaramoorthy, C.; Vigneshwaran, N. Functional finishing in cotton fabrics using zinc oxide nanoparticles. *Bull. Mater. Sci.* **2006**, *29*, 641–645.
30. Vigneshwaran, N.; Kumar, S.; Kathe, A.A.; Varadarajan, P.V.; Prasad, V. Functional finishing of cotton fabrics using zinc oxide soluble starch nanocomposites. *Nanotechnology* **2006**, *17*, 5087–5095.
31. Wang, R.Y.; Zhang, W.; Zhang, L.Y.; Hua, T.; Tang, G.; Peng, X.Q.; Hao, M.H.; Zuo, Q.T. Adsorption characteristics of Cu(II) and Zn(II) by nano-alumina material synthesized by the sol-gel method in batch mode. *Environ. Sci Pollut. Res. Int.* **2019**, *26*, 1595–1605.
32. Council of Europe. *European Pharmacopoeia Commission, European Pharmacopoeia*, 5th ed.; Council of Europe: Strasbourg, France, 2005; pp. 188–191.
33. European Committee for Antimicrobial Susceptibility Testing (EUCAST) of the European Society for Clinical Microbiology and Infectious Diseases (ESCMID). EUCAST Discussion Document, E.Def.5.1. *Clin. Microbiol. Infec.* **2003**, *9*,

34. Peran, J.; Ercegović Ražić, S.; Kosalec, I.; Ziberi, F. Antimicrobial Effectiveness of Cellulose based Fabrics treated with Silver Nitrate Solution using Plasma Processes. *Tekstilec* **2017**, *60*, 247–253.
35. Yan, N.; Zhu, Z.; Jin, L.; Guo, W.; Gan, Y.; Hu, S. Quantitative Characterization of Gold Nanoparticles by Coupling Thin Layer Chromatography with Laser Ablation Inductively Coupled Plasma Mass Spectrometry. *Anal. Chem.* **2015**, *16*, 6079–6087.
36. Yan, N.; Zhu, Z.; He, D.; Jin, L.; Zheng, H.; Hu, S. Simultaneous Determination of Size and Quantification of Gold Nanoparticles by Direct Coupling Thin Layer Chromatography with Catalyzed Luminol Chemiluminescence. *Sci. Rep.* **2016**, *6*, 24577.
37. Elci, S.G.; Yan, B.; Kim, S.T.; Saha, K.; Jiang, Y.; Klemmer, G.A.; Moyano, D.F.; Tonga, G.Y.; Rotello, V.M.; Vachet, R.W. Quantitative imaging of 2 nm monolayer-protected gold nanoparticle distributions in tissues using laser ablation inductively-coupled plasma mass spectrometry (LA-ICP-MS). *Analyst* **2016**, *21*, 2418–2425.
38. Rezić, I.; Ćurković, L.; Ujević, M. Simple methods for characterization of metals in historical textile threads. *Talanta* **2010**, *82*, 237–244.
39. Rezić, I.; Špehar, M.; Jakovljević, S. Characterization of Ag and Au nanolayers on Cu alloys by TLC, SEM-EDS, and ICP-OES. *Mater. Corr.* **2017**, *68*, 560–565.
40. Hodoroaba, V.D.; Motzkus, C.; Macé, T.; Vaslin-Reimann, S. Performance of high-resolution SEM/EDX systems equipped with transmission mode (TSEM) for imaging and measurement of size and size distribution of spherical nanoparticles. *Microsc. Microanal.* **2014**, *20*, 602–612.
41. Reza Mahdavi, S.; Talesh, T.A. The effect of ultrasonic irradiation on the structure, morphology and photocatalytic performance of ZnO nanoparticles by sol-gel method. *Ultrason. Sonochem.* **2017**, *39*, 504–510.
42. Rezić, I.; Majdak, M.; Ljoljić Bilić, V.; Pokrovac, I.; Martinaga, L.; Somogyi Škoc, M.; Kosalec, I. Development of Antibacterial Protective Coatings Active Against MSSA and MRSA on Biodegradable Polymers. *Polymers* **2021**, *13*, 659.
43. Tang, S.; Zheng, J. Antibacterial Activity of Silver Nanoparticles: Structural Effects. *Adv. Health Mater.* **2018**, *7*, 1701503.
44. Li, W.R.; Xie, X.B.; Shi, Q.S.; Duan, S.S.; Ouyang, Y.S.; Chen, Y.B. Antibacterial effect of silver nanoparticles on *Staphylococcus aureus*. *Biometals* **2011**, *24*, 135–141.

45. Mirzajani, F.; Ghassempour, A.; Aliahmadi, A.; Esmaeili, M.A. Antibacterial effect of silver nanoparticles on *Staphylococcus aureus. Res. Microbiol.* **2011**, *162*, 542–549.
46. Grigor'eva A.; Saranina, I.; Tikunova, N.; Safonov, A.; Timoshenko, N.; Rebrov, A.; Ryabchikova, E. Fine mechanisms of the interaction of silver nanoparticles with the cells of *Salmonella typhimurium* and *Staphylococcus aureus. Biometals* **2013**, *26*, 479–488.
47. Martinaga Pintarić, L.; Somogy Škoc, M.; Ljoljić Bilić, V.; Pokrovac, I.; Kosalec, I.; Rezić, I. Synthesis, Modification and Characterization of Antimicrobial Textile Surface Containing ZnO Nanoparticles. *Polymers* **2020**, *12*, 1210.
48. Moore, T.L.; Rodriguez-Lorenzo, L.; Hirsch, V.; Balog, S.; Urban, D.; Jud, C.; Rothen-Rutishauser, B.; Lattuada, M.; Petri-Fink, A. Nanoparticle colloidal stability in cell culture media and impact on cellular interactions. *Chem. Soc. Rev.* **2015**, *44*, 6287–6305.
49. Panáček, A.; Kvítek, L.; Prucek, R.; Kolář, M.; Večeřová, R.; Pizúrová, N.; Zbořil, R. Silver Colloid Nanoparticles: Synthesis, Characterization, and Their Antibacterial Activity. *J. Phys. Chem. B* **2006**, *110*, 16248–16253.
50. Ansari, M.; Khan, H.; Khan, A.; Sultan, A.; Azam, A. Characterization of clinical strains of MSSA, MRSA and MRSE isolated from skin and soft tissue infections and the antibacterial activity of ZnO nanoparticles. *World, J. Microb. Biotechnol.* **2012**, *28*, 1605–1613.
51. Rezić, I.; Steffan, I. ICP-OES determination of metals present in textile materials. *Microchem. J.* **2007**, *85*, 46–51.
52. Rezić, I.; Zeiner, M.; Steffan, I. Determination of 28 selected elements in textiles by axially viewed inductively coupled plasma optical emission spectrometry. *Talanta* **2011**, *83*, 865–871.
53. Özyildiz, F.; Karagönlü, S.; Basal, G.; Uzel, A.; Bayraktar, O. Micro-encapsulation of ozonated red pepper seed oil with antimicrobial activity and application to nonwoven fabric. *Lett. Appl. Microbiol.* **2013**, *56,*168–179.
54. Ramya, K.; Maheshwari, V. Preparation of a naturally driven cotton wound dressing via honey, Tragacanth and Sumac. *Indian, J. Fibre Text. Res.* **2015**, *40*, 213–216.
55. Somogyi Škoc, M.; Macan, J.; Pezelj, E. Modification of polyurethane-coated fabrics by sol-gel thin films. *J. Appl. Pol. Sci.* **2014**, *131*, 39914.
56. Rocha-Selmi, G.A.; Theodoro, A.C.; Thomazini, M.; Bolini, H.M.A.; Favaro-Trindade, C.S. Double emulsion stage prior to complex coacervation process for microencapsulation of sweetener sucralose. *J. Food Eng.* **2013**, *119*, 28–32.

57. He, R.; Ye, J.; Wang, L.; Su, P. Preparation and Evaluation of Microcapsules Encapsulating Royal Jelly Sieve Residue: Flavor and Release Profile. *Appl. Sci.* **2020**, *10*, 8126.
58. Shevtsova, T.; Cavallaro, G.; Lazzara, G.; Milioto, S.; Donchak, V.; Harhay, K.; Korolko, S.; Budkowski, A.; Stetsyshyn, Y. Temperature-responsive hybrid nanomaterials based on modified halloysite nanotubes uploaded with silver nanoparticles. *Coll. Surf. A Physicochem. Eng. Asp.* **2022**, *641*, 128525.
59. Raczkowska, J.; Stetsyshyn, Y.; Awsiuk, K.; Brzychczy-Włoch, M.; Gosiewski, T.; Jany, B.; Lishchynskyi, O.; Shymborska, Y.; Nastyshyn, S.; Bernasik, A.; et al. "Command" surfaces with thermo-switchable antibacterial activity. *Mater. Sci. Eng. C* **2019**, *103*, 109806.
60. Konnova, S.A.; Danilushkina, A.A.; Fakhrullina, G.I.; Akhatova, F.S.; Badrutdinov, A.R.; Fakhrullin, R.F. Silver nanoparticle-coated "cyborg" microorganisms: Rapid assembly of polymer-stabilised nanoparticles on microbial cells. ***RSC Adv.*** **2015**, *5*, 13530–13537.
61. Fries, J.; Getrost, H. *Organic Reagents for Trace Analysis*, 1st ed.; MERCK: Darmstadt, Germany, 1977.
62. Rood, A.S.; McGavran, P.D.; Aanenson, J.W.; Till, J.E. Stochastic estimates of exposure and cancer risk from carbon tetrachloride released to the air from the rocky flats plant. *Risk Anal.* **2001**, *21*, 675–695. https://doi.org/10.1111/0272-4332.214143.
63. Lévesque, B.; Ayotte, P.; Tardif, R.; Ferron, L.; Gingras, S.; Schlouch, E.; Gingras, G.; Levallois, P.; Dewailly, E. Cancer risk associated with household exposure to chloroform. *J. Toxicol. Environ. Health Part. A* **2002**, *65*, 489–502. https://doi.org/10.1080/15287390252807957.

***Funding:** The experimental research[5] which is the foundation of the results presented in this book was funded by the Croatian Science Foundation grant number IP-2019-04-1381 (project under title 'Antibacterial coating for biodegradable medicine materials ABBAMEDICA'). Any opinions, findings and conclusions or recommendations expressed in this material are those of the authors and do not necessarily reflect the views of the Croatian Science Foundation.*

CONCLUDING REMARKS

As we arrive at the culmination of our exploration into the captivating realm of antimicrobial nanoparticles, we find ourselves at a crossroads of scientific achievement and societal responsibility. The journey we undertook through the intricate landscapes of nanotechnology and microbiology has illuminated a path that holds immense promise, tempered by the need for cautious stewardship.

The pages of this book have unveiled the dazzling potential of antimicrobial nanoparticles to transform our approach to infectious diseases. From their ingenious design and synthesis to their remarkable interactions with microbes, we have witnessed the birth of a new era in the ongoing battle against microbial threats. The prospect of overcoming antimicrobial resistance, a challenge that once seemed insurmountable, now glimmers with renewed hope.

Yet, as we celebrate the triumphs and groundbreaking innovations, we must remain ever mindful of the responsibilities that accompany these scientific breakthroughs. The power to manipulate matter at the nanoscale brings with it a profound duty to ensure the judicious and ethical deployment of these technologies. As we harness the capabilities of antimicrobial nanoparticles, we must carefully navigate the potential pitfalls and unintended consequences that may arise.

The pages of this book have also unveiled the multifaceted nature of the journey ahead. The road to realizing the full potential of antimicrobial nanoparticles is paved with challenges – from refining their mechanisms of action and optimizing their delivery, to addressing concerns about safety and environmental impact. These challenges, however, are not insurmountable obstacles, but rather invitations for collaboration and innovation.

The stories of scientists, researchers, and visionaries who have dedicated their lives to unraveling the mysteries of antimicrobial nanoparticles remind us of the boundless capacity of human curiosity and ingenuity. Their tireless efforts inspire us to continue pushing the boundaries of knowledge, fueled by the unwavering belief that science, harnessed for the greater good, can pave the way to a healthier and more resilient future.

As we turn the final page of this book, we find ourselves standing at the threshold of possibility. The journey does not end here; rather, it is a prelude to the next chapter in the evolving narrative of science and discovery. The saga of antimicrobial nanoparticles continues to unfold, inviting new voices, fresh perspectives, and innovative ideas to shape the course of its trajectory.

May the knowledge shared within these pages serve as both a foundation and a catalyst, sparking conversations, inspiring innovations, and guiding us towards a future where the relentless march of microbes is met with the steadfast resolve of human creativity. Let us embrace the challenges and opportunities that lie ahead, driven by the conviction that, united in purpose, we can harness the remarkable potential of antimicrobial nanoparticles to safeguard our health, our communities, and our world.

With gratitude for the journey, we have shared and anticipation for the journeys that await,

Professor Iva Rezić, PhD PhD
August the 10th 2023

ABOUT THE AUTHOR

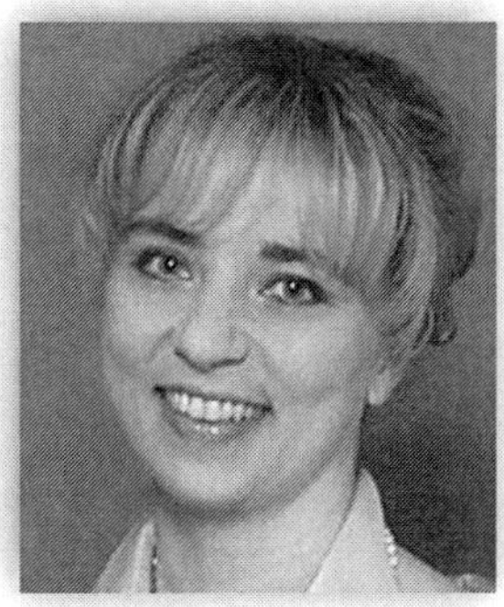

Prof. Iva Rezić PhD PhD was until October 2020 a vice-dean for scientific research at the University of Zagreb, Department of Applied Chemistry, Faculty of Textile Technology, where she led a group of scientists in the field of chemical analysis and material sciences, and taught the courses "Analytical Chemistry," "Instrumental Methods of Analysis," "Physical Chemistry," "Textile Chemistry," and "Computer Method Design of Experiment." She is a double doctor of science laureate: in the field of natural sciences (analytical chemistry) and technical sciences (materials engineering). She applies her professional competences in the management of projects and teams, with a current focus on the development of new materials and the analysis of old precious samples. She has published 56 scientific papers, 3 university and science textbooks, and 5 chapters in scientific books. For her work, she has been awarded with many prizes.